Managing Childhood Medical Emergencies

An Action Guide for Parents and Childcare Providers

Lori Thompson, RN, MA

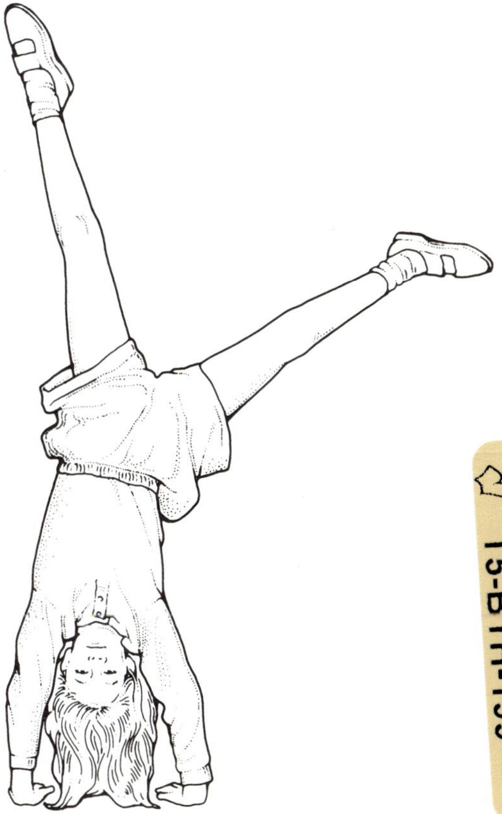

Innovative Learning Publications

Addison-Wesley Publishing Company
Menlo Park, California • Reading, Massachusetts • New York
Don Mills, Ontario • Wokingham, England • Amsterdam
Bonn • Sydney • Singapore • Tokyo • Madrid • San Juan
Paris • Seoul • Milan • Mexico City • Taipei

Acknowledgments

I would like to express thanks to Al Chewning, E.M.T., and fellow Emergency Medical Technicians at the Kempsville Fire Department, Virginia; Grady Tuell, E.M.T.; Steven Thompson, E.M.T.; Stuart Thompson, E.M.T.; Glenn C. Snyders, M.D.; Scott Fisher, M.D.; Neal Katz, M.D.; Ceil Hendrikson, R.N.; the emergency room nurses at Childrens' National Medical Center, Washington, D.C.; Bernadette Lane, R.N., P.N.P.; Marianne Shea, R.N.; Frances Dwyer, R.N., Ph.D.; Patti Rubino, R.N., P.N.P.; Nancy Merrill, R.N., C.N.P.; Elaine Smith, R.N.; Sue Ouillete, R.N., M.N.; Beth Ferguson, R.N.; Glenn Gilbert, Ph.D.; Kenneth Beck, Ph.D.; Catherine Miller, Ph.D.; and the many other health-care professionals consulted for their contributions and review of the material in this manual. Many parents have provided suggestions and guidance, especially Ross and Ettie Mangiapane, Mike and Peggy Riley, Ronnie and Cindi DeConto, Kristin Kulig, Linda Blum, Nancy Madeiros, Brett Smith, Kit and Bette Lawrence, Mike Dwyer, John Lane, Kay Thompson, Don and Evelyn Thompson, Lisa Thompson, Scott and Judy Thompson, and Charlie and Suzie Peckham. Many childcare providers also assisted with review of the material, including David and Sandi Mangiapane and Linda Hanlon. Very special thanks to Tracie Carpenter for her invaluable desktop publishing skills.

The gratitude I feel toward my husband and friend, Steve Thompson, is inexpressible. His patience, understanding, technical assistance, and wonderful sense of humor supported and encouraged me throughout this project.

I am indebted also to my children, Sam and Sara, and to the many other children for whom I have cared, for the inspiration for this manual.

Managing Editor: Cathy Anderson
Project Editor: Martha Siegel
Acquisitions Editor: Lois Fowkes
Production/Mfg: Leanne Collins
Design Manager: Jeff Kelly
Cover/Text Design: Lisa Raine
Art Manager: Rachel Gage
Illustrators: Molly Babich, Conery Calhoon, Gale Mueller, Brian Evans
Cover Illustration: Cindy Wooley

This book is published by Innovative Learning Publications™, an imprint of the Alternative Publishing Group of Addison-Wesley Publishing Company.

ISBN 0-201-49050-1

CONTENTS

- Experiencing lips, gums, or nails that are pale or a bluish color.

Treat signs of breathing difficulty as needed. See **Breathing Difficulty—General,** page 71.

5. If the child is not breathing, see **Rescue Breathing/ Cardiopulmonary Resuscitation (CPR):** 0–1 year, page 27; 1–8 years, page 33; 8+ years, page 39.

Checking Temperature

There are three places to take a child's temperature: under the tongue (oral method), in the rectum (rectal method), and in the armpit (axillary method). There are many blood vessels in each of these areas. When the thermometer lays against the blood vessels, the heat of the blood makes the mercury inside the thermometer rise.

The child's temperature will be slightly different in each of these three locations. The rectal temperature measures the heat deep inside the child's body, so the measurement may be about 1 degree higher than if you take the temperature orally, and it may be about 2 degrees higher than if you take the temperature under the arm. However, this varies.

Where you take the child's temperature depends on: 1) her age; 2) whether or not she is unconscious; 3) whether or not she is cooperative (she may fight the procedure, may be extremely upset, or may be mentally retarded or developmentally delayed and not able to understand and follow instructions); and, 4) the doctor's preference (many doctors prefer a rectal measurement because it is the best indicator of the child's "true" temperature). Other factors may also play a part. The charts below give guidelines for when to use each method.

Range of Normal Temperatures

Oral	97.6°–98.6°F
Axillary	97°–98°F
Rectal	99°–99.6°F

Note: Everyone's body temperature is higher with activity, is lowest in the morning, and is highest in the late afternoon.

Using a Digital Thermometer

The preceding instructions are for glass and mercury thermometers. You may choose to take a child's temperature with a digital thermometer instead. (Figure 9)

Digital thermometers are as accurate as glass thermometers but are safer to use and easier to read. They also register temperature much more quickly; most models display the final reading within 30 seconds to 1 minute. Most have a plastic body about the size of a pen, and can be used for the oral, rectal, or axillary methods. They display the figures, such as 99.6°F, in a window and beep when the final temperature has been reached. Insertion techniques are the same as for a glass thermometer, but some models have a probe cover for sanitary purposes. Check the available models for ease of use and for different warranties.

A digital thermometer requires a battery for use, so it is a good idea to have extra batteries on hand and a glass thermometer available as a backup if the batteries fail.

Figure 9

digital thermometer

Using an Ear Thermometer

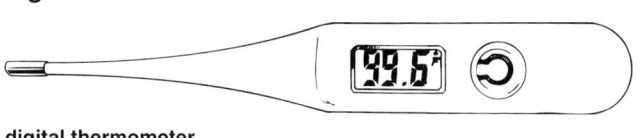

The newest type of thermometer for home use is the ear thermometer. (Figure 10) Ear thermometers are most commonly used in pediatricians' offices. When correctly inserted into the ear, the thermometer takes an infrared "snapshot" of the energy given off by the eardrum. The thermometer then converts this "snapshot" into a numerical value, the equivalent of an oral or rectal temperature.

The energy from the eardrum is a good indicator of body temperature because the same blood vessel that supplies the eardrum also supplies the body's thermostat in the brain. The thermostat senses whether body temperature is high or low and stimulates the body to make necessary adjustments.

Figure 10

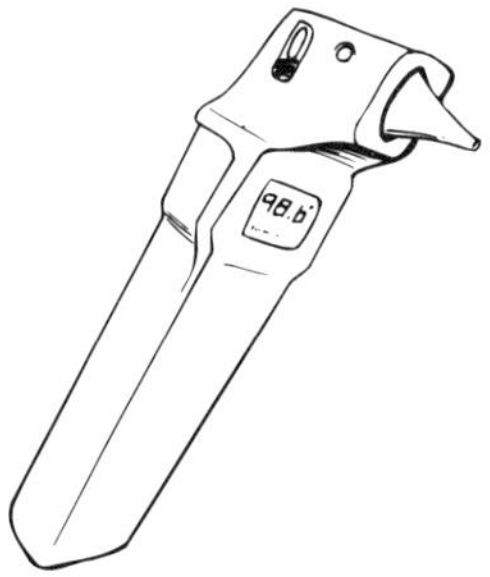

ear thermometer

Step 2: Is the Child Breathing?

To check

a. Open the airway. See **Rescue Breathing/Cardiopulmonary Resuscitation (CPR):** 0–1 year, page 27; 1–8 years, page 33; 8+ years, page 39.

If you do not suspect a back or neck injury: lift the child's chin up gently with one hand while pushing down on the forehead to tilt the head back with the other. Tilt an infant's head back only enough so the corner of the mouth is in line with the middle section of the ear. Tilt a child's head slightly farther back so the teeth are almost brought together. The neck should not be overextended or stretched far back.

If the possibility of a back or neck injury exists, use the jaw-thrust technique: place two or three fingers on each side of the lower jaw and lift upward.

b. Look at the child's chest for movement. (With an infant, look at the abdomen as well.)

c. Place your face next to the child's mouth and nose—listen and feel for air.

d. Check for 3–5 seconds.

Yes

Proceed to Step 4.

Yes, but with difficulty

a. Make sure the airway is open.

b. If the child is conscious and you do not suspect a back or neck injury, sit the child in an upright position, supporting her head and shoulders.

c. **Call 911 or the rescue squad** if you have not already done so.

d. Observe. If breathing stops, see **Rescue Breathing/Cardiopulmonary Resuscitation (CPR):** 0–1 year, page 27; 1–8 years, page 33; 8+ years, page 39.

e. Proceed to Step 4.

No

a. Give two rescue breaths. See **Rescue Breathing/Cardiopulmonary Resuscitation (CPR):** 0–1 year, page 27; 1–8 years, page 33; 8+ years, page 39.

b. Proceed to Step 3.

b. If there is a possibility of a back or neck injury, do not bend his neck or tilt his head back. Place two or three fingers under each side of his lower jaw and lift upward (jaw-thrust technique). (Figure 4)

5. Check the infant's breathing.

Look at his chest; listen and feel for air from his mouth or nose. Check for 3–5 seconds. (Figure 5)

If the infant is breathing but not responsive,

a. Position his head to keep the airway open. Use the jaw-thrust technique if there is a possibility of a back or neck injury.

b. If a back or neck injury is not suspected, place the infant in the recovery position, as follows:

1. Kneel beside the infant.
2. Turn the infant onto his side by pulling him toward you.
3. Position his head to keep the airway open.
4. Support the infant's body by placing rolled-up clothing or a small blanket along his torso, or hold him in position while an assistant summons help. (Figure 6)

c. Call 911 or the rescue squad.

d. Return to the infant and await medical assistance. Continue to observe his breathing. If breathing stops, follow instructions below.

If the infant is not breathing, give two rescue breaths.

a. Cover the infant's mouth and nose tightly with your mouth.

b. Give two slow, shallow breaths. Give only enough air

Figure 4

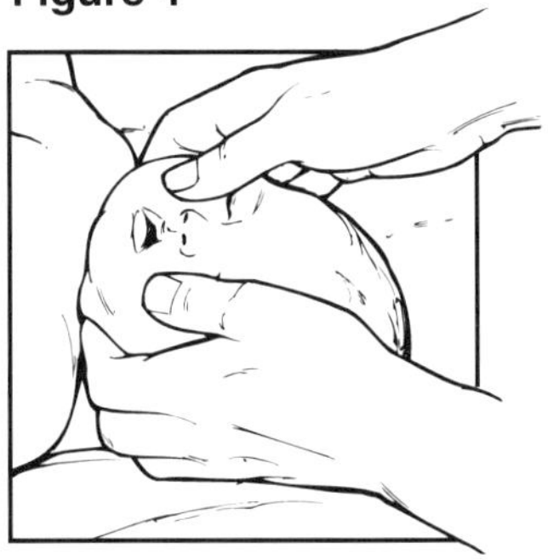

Figure 5

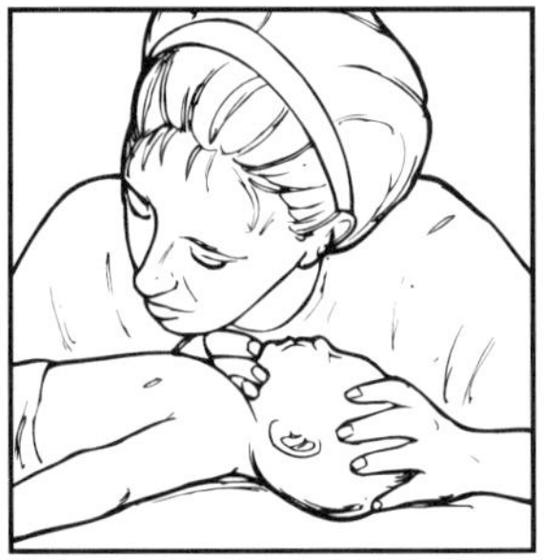

Figure 6

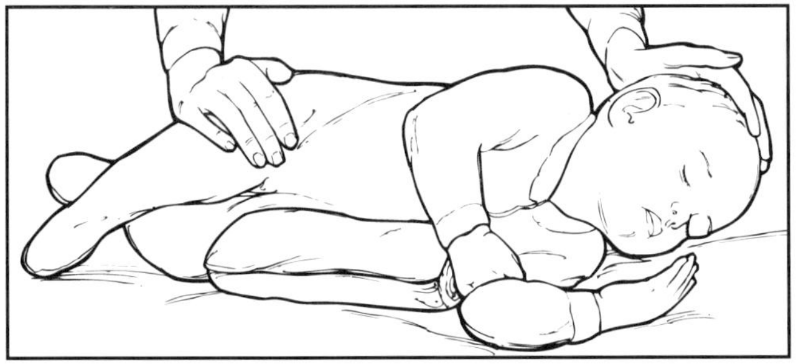

If there is no pulse and no breathing, continue CPR until medical help arrives or breathing and pulse return.

(Figure 14)

Recheck the infant's breathing and pulse every few minutes. Continue CPR, or rescue breathing, as necessary.

Figure 14

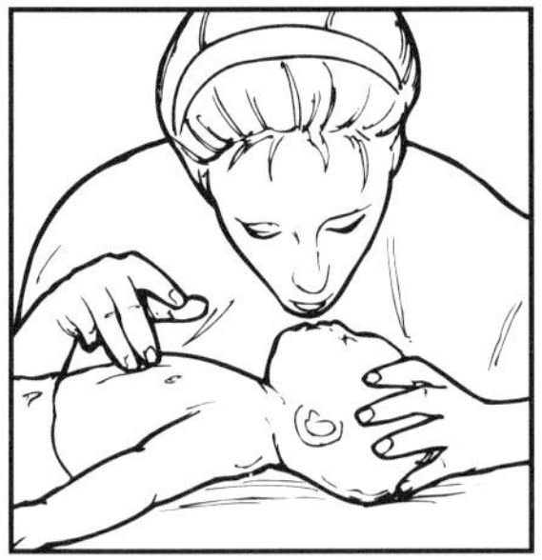

If a pulse is present but the child is still not breathing, continue rescue breathing. Give one breath every 3 seconds.

a. Count "1-and-2-and-3-and," breathe, count "1-and-2-and-3-and," breathe, and so on. (Figure 9)

b. Perform rescue breathing for 1 minute, then recheck breathing.

c. If you are alone, **call 911 or the rescue squad** now.

d. Return to the child, and recheck breathing and pulse.

e. Continue rescue breathing until medical help arrives or the child begins breathing on her own. Recheck breathing every few minutes during rescue breathing.

Figure 9

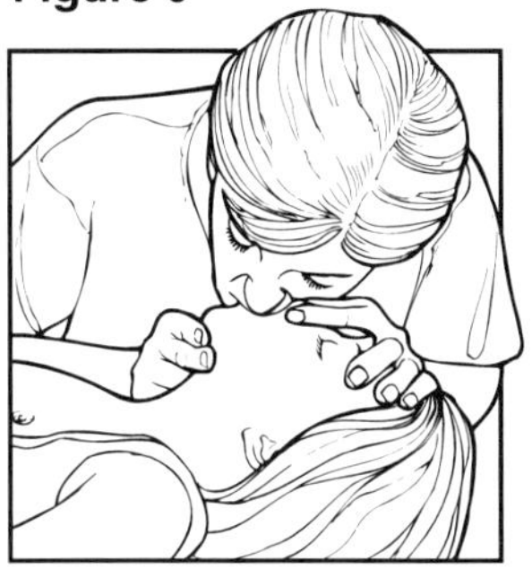

If there is no pulse, find the location for chest compressions.

a. With the first two fingers of your left hand (your right hand if you are left-handed), find the bottom of the child's rib cage. Slide your fingers upward along the rib cage until you feel the tip of the breastbone in the center of the chest. Place the heel of your right hand next to your two fingers, higher on the breast bone. (Figure 10) Remove your two fingers from the child's chest. The heel of your hand should not be on the breastbone tip because you might break it. The fingers of your right hand should be pointing toward the child's arm. Raise your fingers up, off the chest.

b. Put your other hand on the child's forehead to hold her head still and to keep the airway open through out CPR. You also will use this hand to pinch her nose shut when giving a breath.

Figure 10

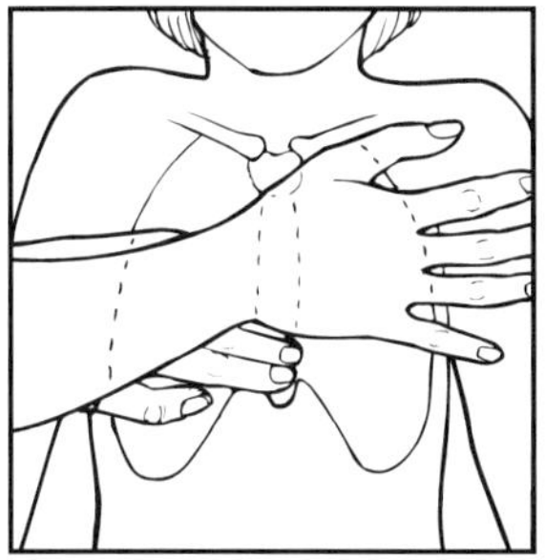

3. Position the child on his back.

a. Place the child on his back on a firm, flat surface. (Figure 3)

b. If there is a possibility of a back or neck injury, see **Back and Neck Injuries,** page 45, for positioning.

c. Open the child's clothing to reveal his chest.

4. Open the airway.

a. If you do not suspect a back or neck injury, lift the child's chin up gently with one hand while pushing down on his forehead with your other hand. Tip his head back so his chin is pointing toward the ceiling. (Figure 4)

b. If there is a possibility of a back or neck injury, do not bend his neck or tilt his head back. Place two or three fingers under each side of his lower jaw and lift upward (jaw-thrust technique). (Figure 5)

5. Check the child's breathing.

Look at his chest; listen and feel for air from his mouth or nose. Check for 3–5 seconds. (Figure 6)

If the child is breathing but not responsive,

a. Position his head to keep the airway open. Use the jaw-thrust technique if there is a possibility of a back or neck injury.

b. If a back or neck injury is not suspected, place the child in the recovery position, as follows:

1. Kneel beside the child.
2. Turn the child onto his side by pulling him toward you.
3. Position the child's head to keep the airway open.
4. Support his body by bending the arm and leg

Figure 3

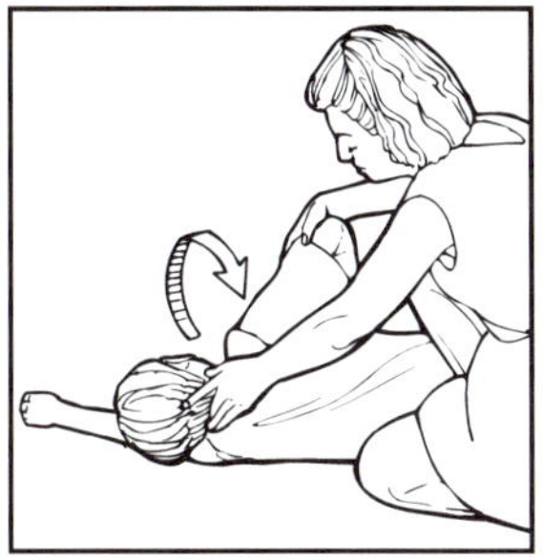

Figure 4

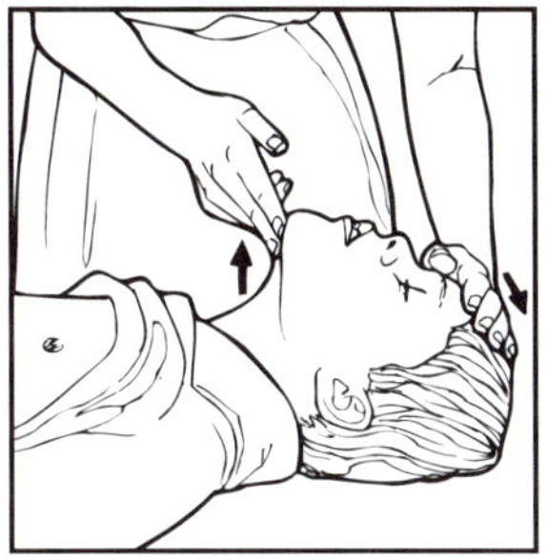

Figure 5

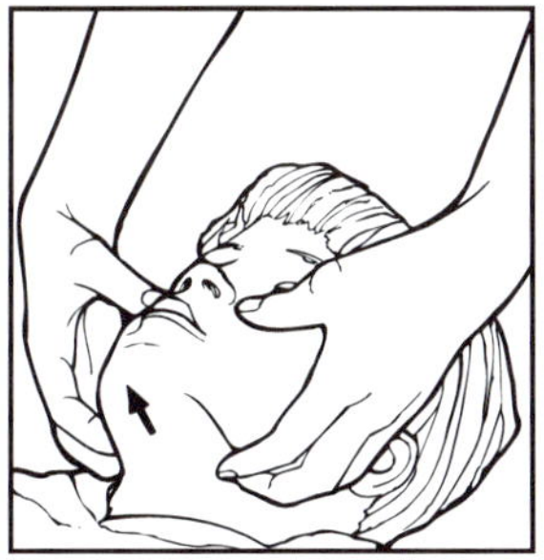

Figure 6

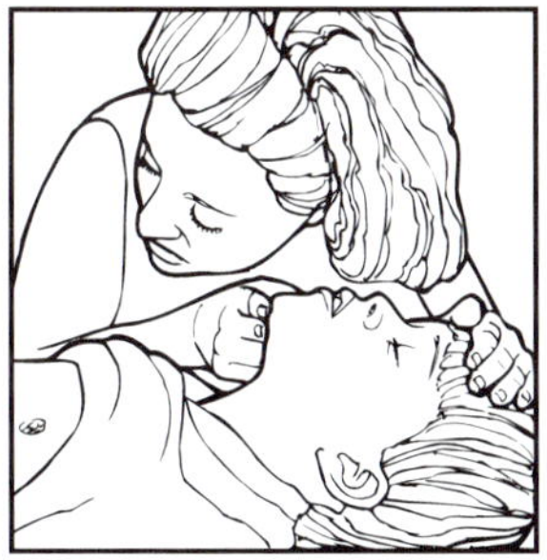

Figure 7

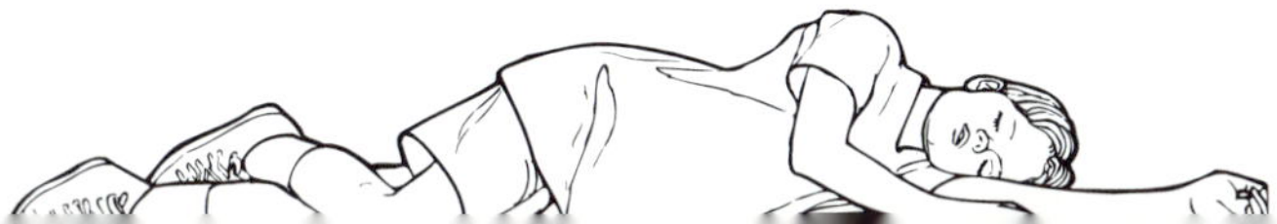

If there is a pulse but no breathing, continue rescue breathing at the rate of one breath every 5 seconds until medical help arrives or breathing returns.

(Figure 15)

Recheck the child's breathing every few minutes. Stop rescue breathing if he breathes on his own, but continue to observe.

Figure 15

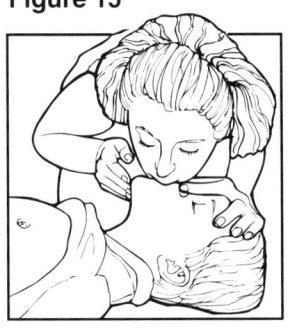

If there is no pulse and no breathing, continue CPR until medical help arrives or breathing and pulse return.

(Figure 16)

Recheck the child's breathing and pulse every few minutes. Continue CPR, or rescue breathing, as necessary.

Figure 16

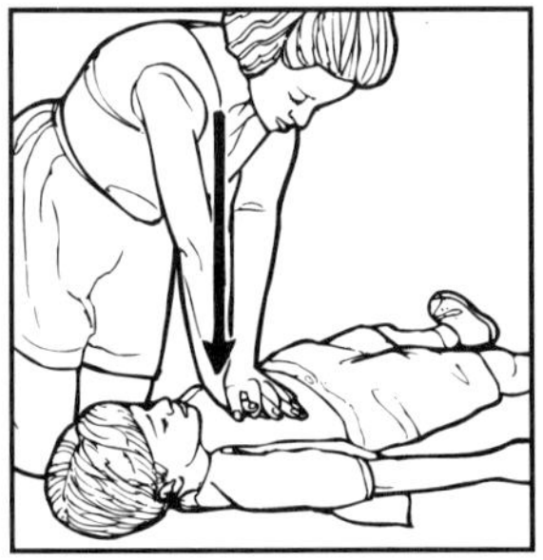

Follow the instructions below, keeping in mind these principles:

- Do not bend or twist the child's neck or body—movement may put pressure on the spinal cord or cause a broken bone to damage it.
- Keep the child's head, neck, and body in line, and support them all. If you must roll the child, keep his head in the position in which you found it.
- Use more than one person to move the child, if possible.

If the Child Is in Danger

If the Child Is Face Down and You Are Alone

Stoop down at the child's head. Grasp his shoulders and support his head firmly between your forearms. Cautiously drag the child away from danger. (Figure 6)

If the Child Is Face Down and You Have Help

Follow these instructions if a blanket, coat, board, or ironing board is available; if not available, follow the instructions above. Use at least three people—one to support the child's head in the position found, one at his shoulders, and at least one to support his waist and legs. (Figure 7) The person positioned at the head should count and give the command to roll the child onto his side. Roll him as a unit while keeping him straight. Slide a blanket, coat, or board next to the child and then roll him as a unit onto his back on top of the blanket, coat, or board. (Figure 8) Carry the child to safety. Keep his head and neck well supported at all times.

If the Child Is on His Back and You Are Alone

Stand behind the child's head. Grasp under his shoulders, at the shoulder blades. Support his head with your forearms; drag him to safety. (Figure 9)

Figure 6

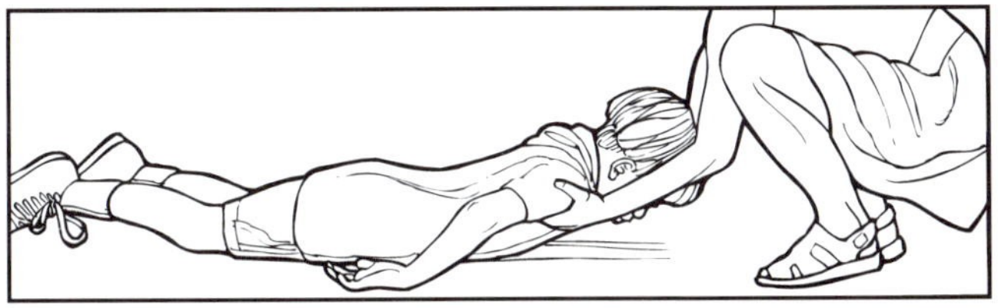

Figure 7

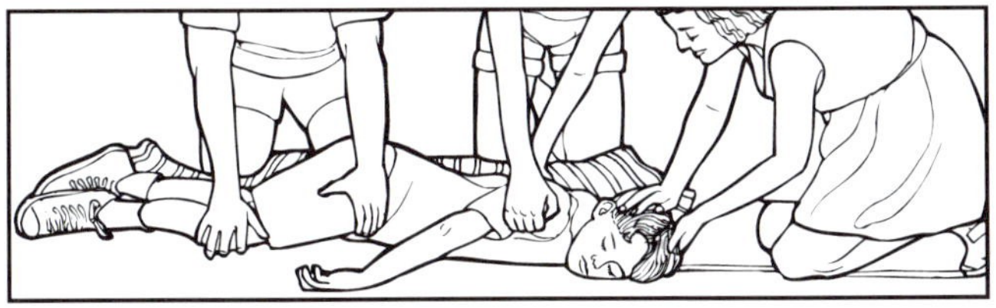

Figure 8

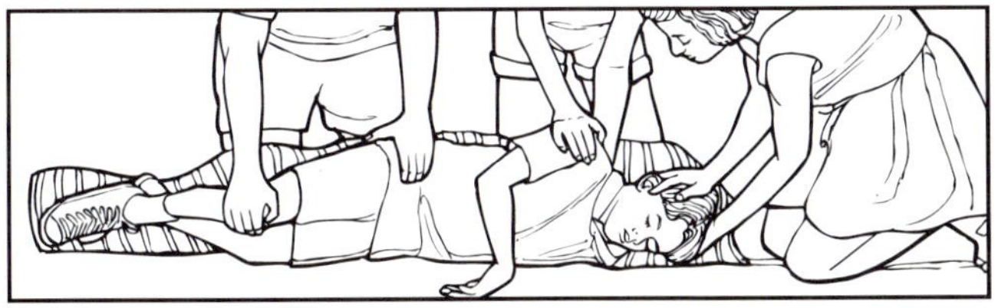

Figure 9

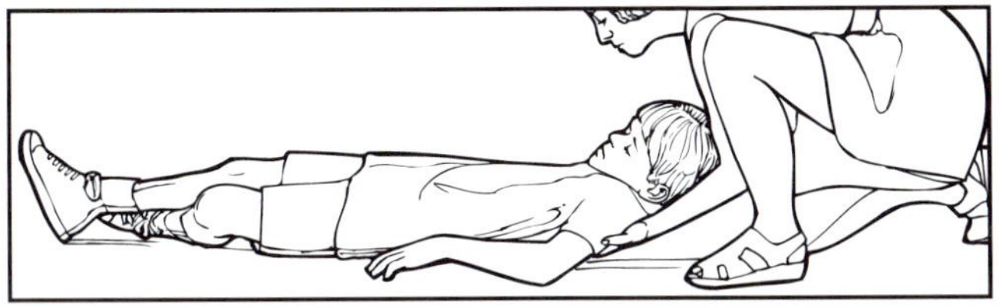

Home Treatment

If the child does not have to see a doctor immediately, do the following:

1. Keep the wound clean and dry; change the dressing daily or when soiled or wet.
2. Check the wound daily for signs of infection. (The wound may be red, hot, tender, swollen; it may have pus; or the child may have fever.) If an infection is present, see the doctor to have the wound examined. A severe infection may develop after a human bite because the human mouth contains many bacteria.
3. Notify the doctor if the animal develops rabies. If the animal is alive and healthy after two weeks, it does not have rabies and therefore did not pass rabies to the child.

Once the most life-threatening problems have been attended to, you may proceed with further treatment as indicated in the following instructions.

2. Slow the flow of venom.

a. Remove the bee stinger, if present. Honeybees usually leave the stinger, whereas wasps (hornets, yellow jackets) and bumblebees do not. They may, however, sting repeatedly. Do not squeeze the stinger—it will release more venom if you do. Use the edge of a razor, knife, or fingernail to scrape the stinger off sideways. (Figure 3)

b. Keep the affected limb down, below the level of the heart.

c. Wash the affected area vigorously with soap and cold water.

d. Apply ice, wrapped in cloth or plastic, to the area. (Figure 4)

Figure 3

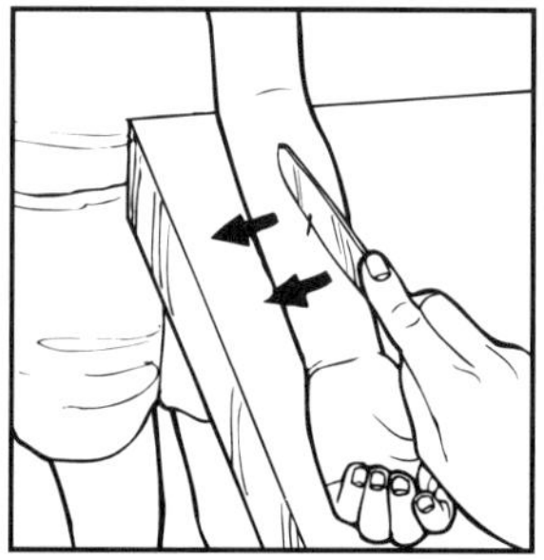

Figure 4

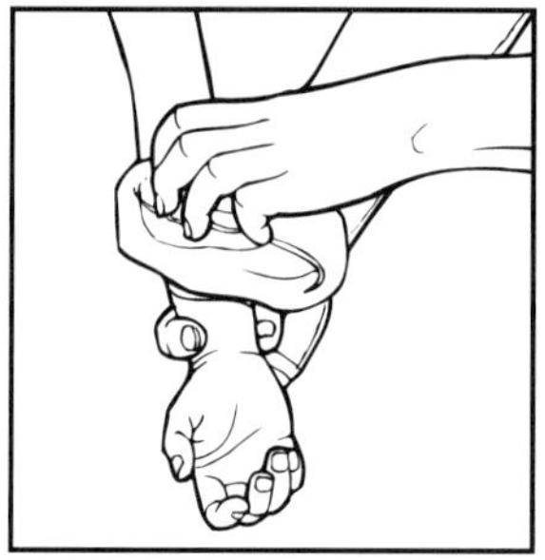

3. Seek medical assistance.

a. If you have not already called 911 or the rescue squad, take the child to the nearest medical facility if any of these symptoms develop: breathing difficulty, facial swelling, nausea, abdominal cramps, muscle cramps, sweating, or fainting.

b. While on the way to the medical facility, keep ice on the affected area.

c. While on the way to the medical facility, keep the child in an upright position.

2. Follow the appropriate instructions as follows.

- If the answers to both of these questions are *no,* follow the instructions as indicated in **If No Fracture Is Suspected,** below.
- If the answer to either of these questions is *yes,* follow the instructions as indicated in **If a Fracture Is Suspected,** below.
- If the child is bleeding from the mouth or into the throat, follow the instructions as indicated in **If Bleeding is From the Mouth or Into the Throat,** page 68.

If No Fracture Is Suspected

1. Stop the flow of blood.

a. Apply direct pressure. Press firmly on the wound with sterile gauze or a clean cloth. (Figure 2) For a nose-bleed, pinch the nostrils together.

b. Raise the injured limb higher than the heart unless doing so causes pain. Support the limb, as necessary. (Figure 3)

c. Continue to press firmly until the bleeding stops. Do not remove the cloth, and add more layers as necessary. (Removing the cloth may restart the bleeding.)

d. If the bleeding does not slow down within 5 minutes, press more firmly.

If the bleeding does not slow down within 5 more minutes, or if there is a rapid flow or large amount of bleeding,

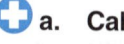

a. Call 911 or the rescue squad.

Figure 2

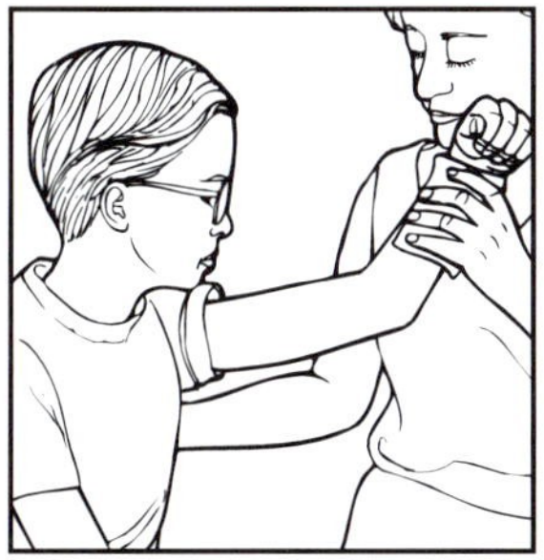

Figure 3

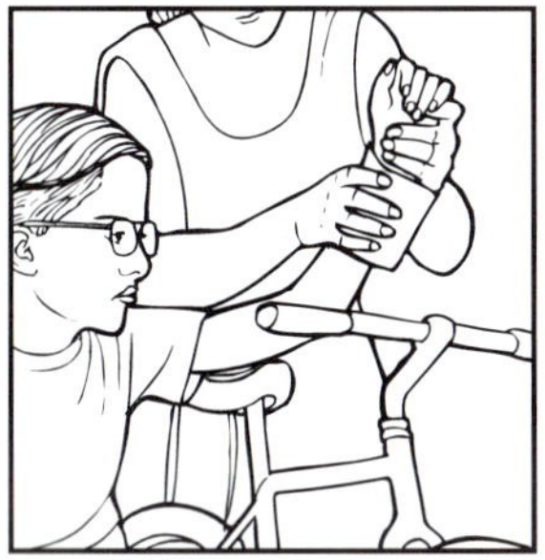

If Bleeding Cannot Be Immediately Controlled: Body or Head Wounds

1. Apply direct pressure to the wound.

Continue to press firmly on the wound (if no fracture is suspected), until medical help arrives. Be sure to press gently if the wound is on the child's head. (Figure 10)

Figure 10

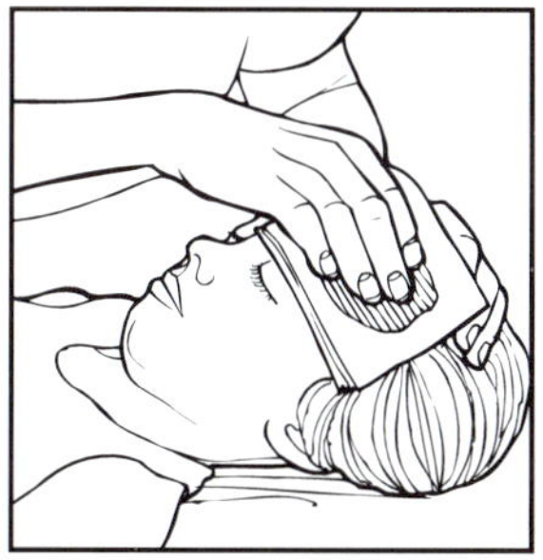

2. Treat for shock.

See **Shock,** page 169.

If Bleeding Is From the Mouth or Into the Throat

1. Position the child.

Position the child on her side so blood can drain from her mouth. (Figure 11)

NOTE: *If a back or neck injury is suspected, see* ***Back and Neck Injuries,*** *page 45, for proper positioning.*

Figure 11

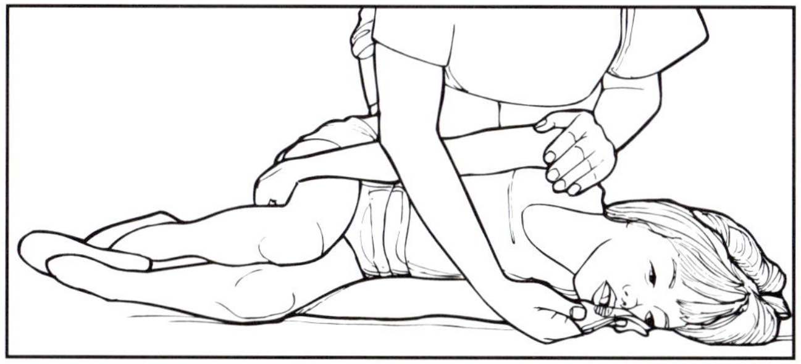

2. Keep the airway open.

a. Position the child's head so her chin is not resting on her chest, blocking the airway. (Figure 12)

b. Clear the child's mouth of blood, tooth fragments, or other material.

Figure 12

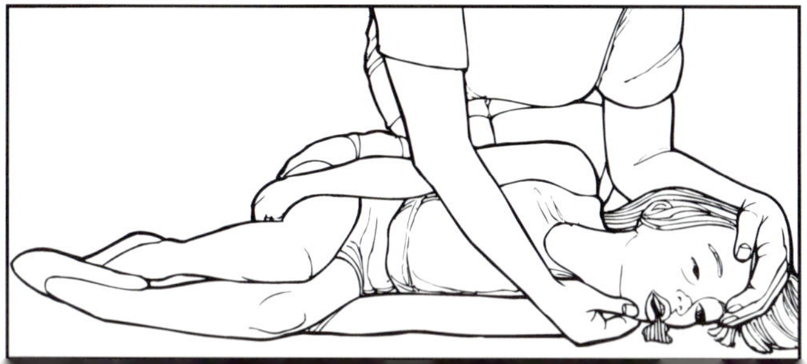

3. Call 911 or the rescue squad for rapid or large amount of bleeding.

4. Treat for shock.

See **Shock,** page 169.

Safety Highlights

Do

- **Do** act calmly to prevent anxiety in and greater breathing difficulty for the child.
- **Do** sit the child in an upright position to ease breathing.
- **Do** consider the possibility of a foreign object in the airway if the attack came on suddenly and the child was eating or normally puts "everything" in his or her mouth, and if the child cannot cry or speak.

Don't

- **Don't** give the child any medications to relieve breathing difficulty unless instructed to do so by the doctor.
- **Don't** allow the child to stand too close to the hot water when giving him or her a steam treatment; the water or steam may burn the skin.

Immediate Action

1. Check for signs of breathing difficulty.

The child is

- Breathing much more rapidly than usual (0–1 year—more than sixty times per minute; 1+ years—more than forty times per minute). Count breaths per minute when the child is at rest. Try to calm him or distract him, and then count.
- Pulling in his chest and/or stomach muscles so deeply that you can see his ribs much more easily than usual.
- Looking very anxious with trouble breathing, or telling you he is having trouble breathing.
- Having difficulty swallowing, which is causing drooling, and breathing with his mouth wide open and his chin jutting forward.
- Breathing noisily.
- Experiencing hoarseness with a cough that sounds like a barking seal.
- Experiencing a congested cough, and there is a "rattling" feeling when you feel his chest or back.

2. Keep the child's nasal passages clear. Help the child clear her nose. If the child is an infant or toddler, use a bulb syringe or aspirator.
3. Monitor the child's temperature. Treat fever over 101°F as recommended in **Fever,** page 125, or according to the doctor's instructions.
4. Consult the child's doctor for recommendations about children's cold medicines and the use of a vaporizer, and if there is increased breathing difficulty.

If the Child Has Previously Been Treated for Asthma

If the child has never been treated for asthma, see **If the Child Has Not Been Treated for Asthma Before,** page 78. If the child has been treated for asthma in the past, do the following:

1. Give the child her prescribed medication for asthma attacks.

Follow the doctor's instructions to administer the child's asthma medication. (Figure 3) If you are not the child's parent or legal guardian, do not medicate the child. Contact the child's parent, guardian, or doctor.

Figure 3

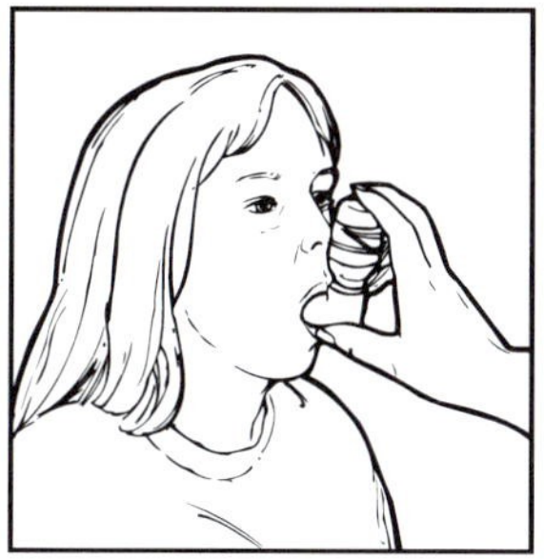

2. Maximize the child's breathing ability.

a. Sit the child in an upright position. Help the child choose a comfortable position; many children prefer to lean foward, supporting their weight on a table or chair.

b. Do not give the child anything to drink.

3. Reduce the child's anxiety.

a. Speak and act in a calm manner. Anxiety can cause the child's airways to narrow.

b. Keep the child calm and quiet. Use slow-breathing techniques, inhaling deeply through the nose, holding the breath, and breathing out through pursed lips as if blowing out candles. Have the child look at you and breathe as slowly and deeply as she can. Breathe with the child for as long as she will cooperate.

c. Keep the child's environment quiet.

Immediate Action

1. Stop skin tissue from burning.

a. Cover flames with a blanket or roll the child on the ground. (Figure 1)

b. Put the burned area into cold water or apply clean, cold, wet cloths to the area immediately. (Figures 2, 3)

c. Leave the cold cloths on or keep the burned area in cold water for at least 5 minutes. If the burn is large (larger than the size of the child's hand), do not immerse the burned area in cold water for longer than 10 minutes—the child's body temperature may become too cool.

2. Look at the burn to identify the type of burn.

Determine whether the burn is first, second, or third degree.

First degree The skin is smooth, red, and painful, but *not* broken. (Sunburn is an example.)

Second degree Several layers of skin may have been burned; the area is red or purplish; blisters may appear; there is pain and some swelling.

Third degree The skin has a white or grayish appearance; all skin layers have been destroyed. The tissue under the skin can be seen; there is no pain because nerve endings have been destroyed.

3. Follow the appropriate instructions as follows, depending on the type and location of the burn.

If you cannot decide whether a burn is second or third degree, treat it as if it were third degree.

Figure 1

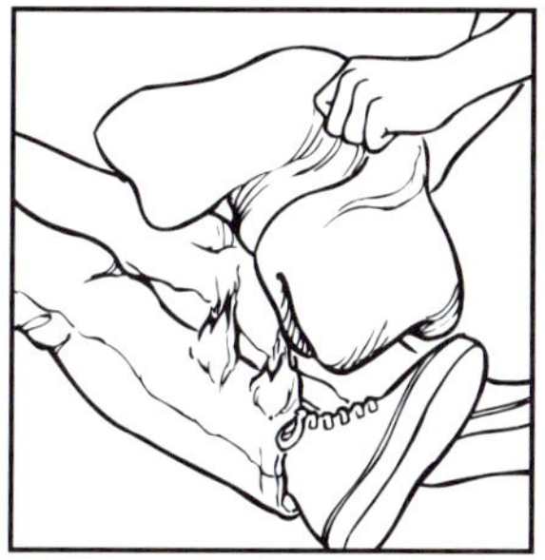

Figure 2

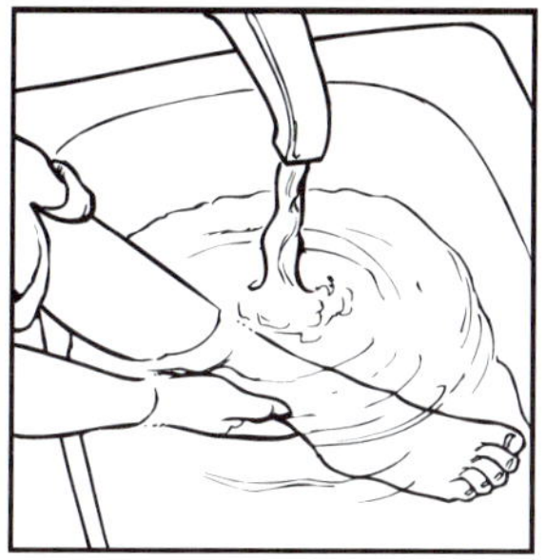

Figure 3

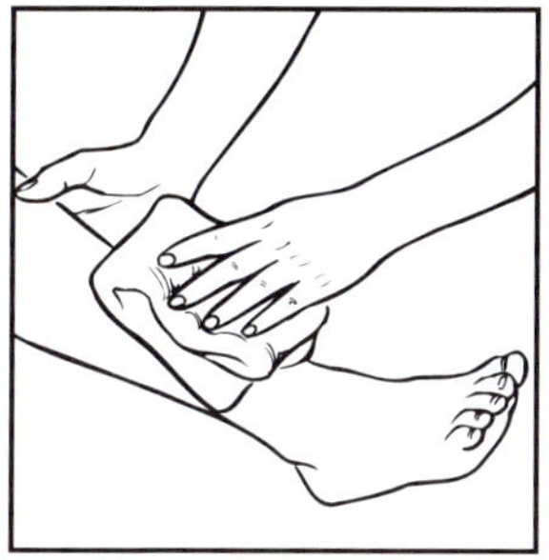

b. Cover the burned area with a sterile gauze dressing; a smooth, clean cloth (for example, a torn sheet or pillowcase); or plastic food wrap. Or, for large, extensive burns, wrap the child in a clean sheet or cloth or in plastic wrap. (Figures 8, 9) To prevent suffocation, do not place plastic wrap over the child's face.

3. Reduce the swelling.

a. If the burn involves the face, or if the child was exposed to smoke or hot gases, sit the child in an upright position.

b. If an arm or leg is burned, raise it higher than the heart. (Figure 10)

c. Apply a clean, cold, wet pack, wrapped in plastic, over the burned area. Leave the pack on for 5–10 minutes. Remove the pack if the area becomes numb. (Figure 11)

4. Observe breathing.

a. If breathing becomes difficult, keep the child in an upright position. Tilt the child's head back to keep the airway open.

b. Keep both the child and the environment calm and quiet—anxiety can cause the child's airways to become narrow.

c. If the child becomes unconscious, check for breathing. If the child is not breathing, begin rescue breathing. See **Rescue Breathing/Cardiopulmonary Resuscitation (CPR):** 0–1 year, page 27; 1–8 years, page 33; 8+ years, page 39.

5. Treat for shock.

See **Shock,** page 169. Do not lie the child down if the face or neck is burned.

Figure 8

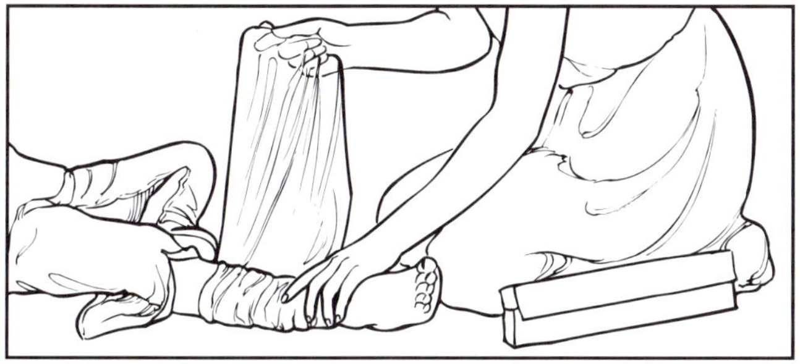

Figure 9

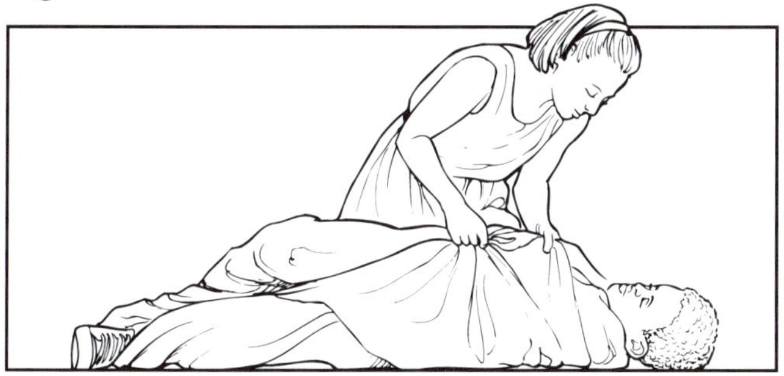

Figure 10

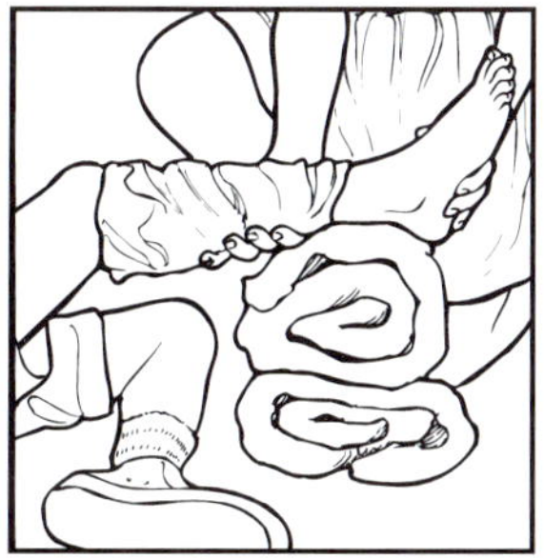

Figure 11

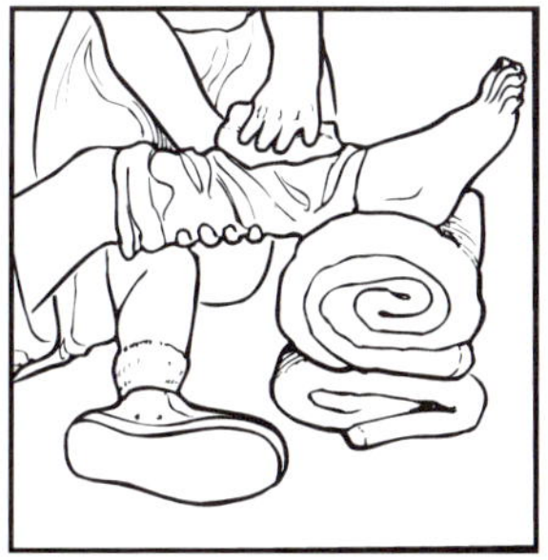

- There is a gradual loss of color—the skin around the mouth and the lips, gums, and nails may become blue.
- The infant pulls in his chest deeply in an attempt to breathe.
- The infant may lose consciousness. See **If the Choking Infant Is Unconscious (Not Responsive),** page 95, if this happens.

2. If the infant seems to be choking, position the infant face down.

a. Place the infant face down along the length of your forearm (the infant's jaw should rest in your fingers).

b. Lower your arm—the infant's head should be lower than his feet.

c. Hold the infant against your body or thigh for extra support. Hold his head firmly.

3. Give five back blows.

Using the heel of your free hand, give five forceful back blows, high on the infant's back, between the shoulder blades. (Figure 1)

Figure 1

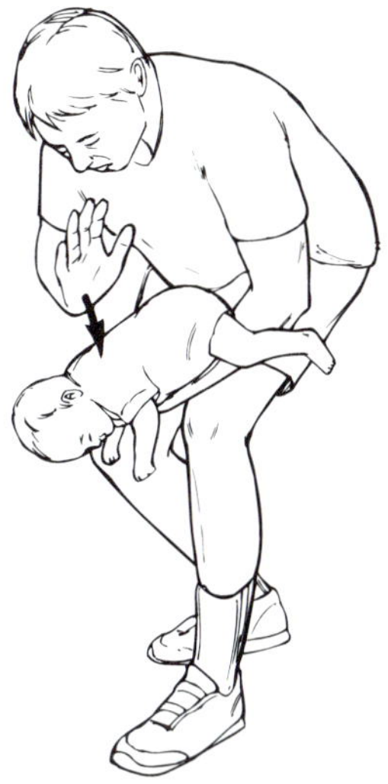

4. If the object on which the infant is choking has not become dislodged, reposition the infant face up.

a. Sandwich the infant between your arms and turn the infant onto his back, along the length of your forearm.

b. Lower your arm—the infant's head should be lower than his feet. (Figure 2)

Figure 2

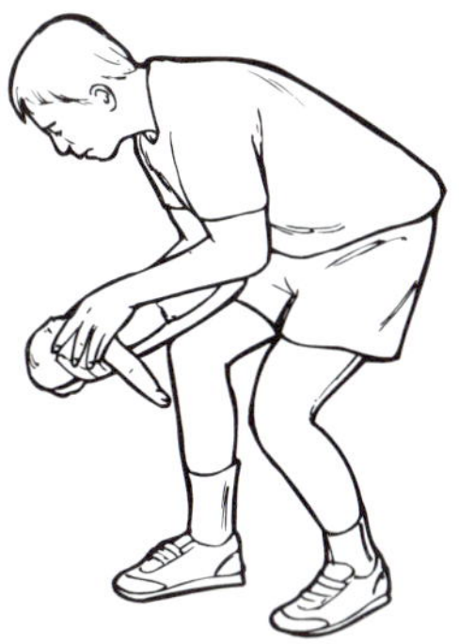

5. Find the correct finger placement for chest thrusts.

a. Place your ring finger on the infant's breastbone at the level of the nipples. Point toward the infant's arm.

If the infant is not breathing,

proceed to Step 6.

If the infant is breathing but is not responsive:

Figure 10

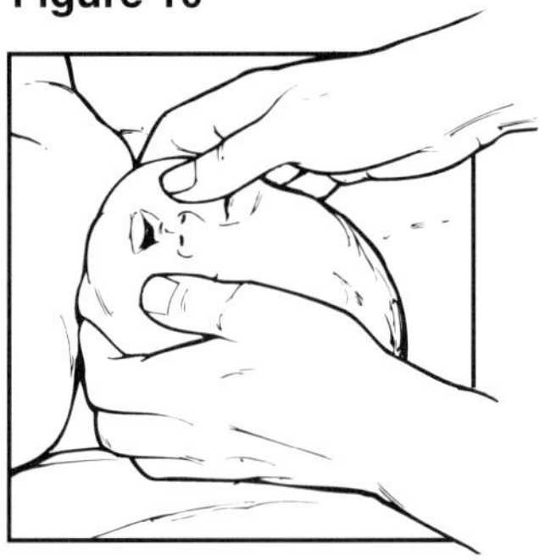

a. Position his head to keep the airway open. Use the jaw-thrust technique if there is a possibility of a back or neck injury. (Figure 10)

b. If a back or neck injury is not suspected, place the infant in the recovery position, as follows:

   1. Kneel beside the infant.
   2. Turn the infant onto his side by pulling him toward you.
   3. Position his head to keep the airway open.
   4. Support the infant's body by placing rolled-up clothing or a small blanket along his torso, or hold him in position if help has been summoned.

c. If help has not yet been summoned, **call 911 or the rescue squad** now.

d. Return to the infant and await medical assistance. Continue to observe his breathing. If breathing stops, proceed to Step 6, below.

6. Give two rescue breaths.

Figure 11

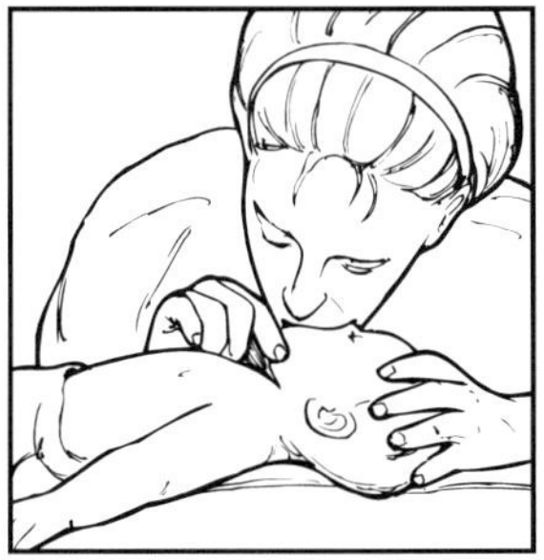

a. Leaving your hand on the infant's forehead, tightly cover the infant's mouth and nose with your mouth. (Figure 11)

b. Gently blow into the infant's mouth for 1 to $1\frac{1}{2}$ seconds, pause, and then give a second breath for 1 to $1\frac{1}{2}$ seconds.

c. Look at or feel the infant's chest when giving a breath—the chest should rise as the lungs fill with air.

d. If you feel resistance, as if the breath did not go in

18. Repeat Steps 8–15 until:

- The object is dislodged. Proceed to Step 19.
- The infant regains consciousness.
- Medical help arrives.

19. Check breathing.

If the obstruction is removed and the infant is breathing, see **When to See a Doctor,** page 101.

If the infant is not crying or if you are not sure if the infant is breathing:

a. Position the infant on his back.

b. Open the airway:

1. Place one hand on the infant's forehead.

2. Place the fingers of your other hand on the bony part of the lower jaw.

3. Tilt the infant's head back. The middle of the back of his head should be flat, and the corner of his mouth should be in line with his earlobe.

4. Keep your hand on the infant's forehead to keep the airway open.

c. Place your ear over the infant's mouth and look at his chest. Look, listen, and feel for a breath for 3–5 seconds. (Figure 19)

d. If the infant is not breathing, see **Rescue Breathing/ Cardiopulmonary Resuscitation (CPR),** page 27. If the obstruction is removed and the infant is breathing, see **When to See a Doctor,** page 101.

Figure 19

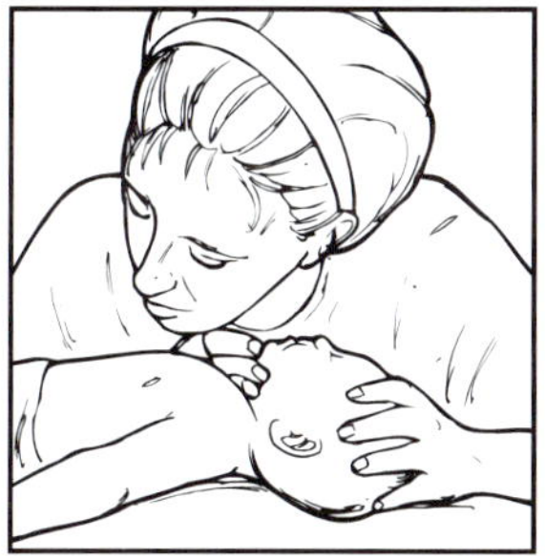

- There is a gradual loss of color—the skin around the mouth and the lips, gums, and nails may become blue.
- The child pulls in her chest deeply in an attempt to breathe.
- The child may lose consciousness. See **If the Choking Child Is Unconscious (Not Responsive),** page 106, if this happens.

2. If the child seems to be choking, position the child for abdominal thrusts.

Stand behind the child and wrap your arms around her waist.

3. Find the correct hand placement for abdominal thrusts.

a. Place the thumb of one fist in the middle of the child's abdomen, slightly above the navel (belly-button) and below the rib cage. (Figure 1)

b. Place your other hand on top of your fist.

4. Give five abdominal thrusts.

a. Press inward and upward toward the child's chest. Pause for 1 second between thrusts. Each thrust is an attempt to force out of the windpipe the object that is causing the child to choke. (Figure 2)

b. Adjust the force of the thrusts to the size of the child.

Figure 1

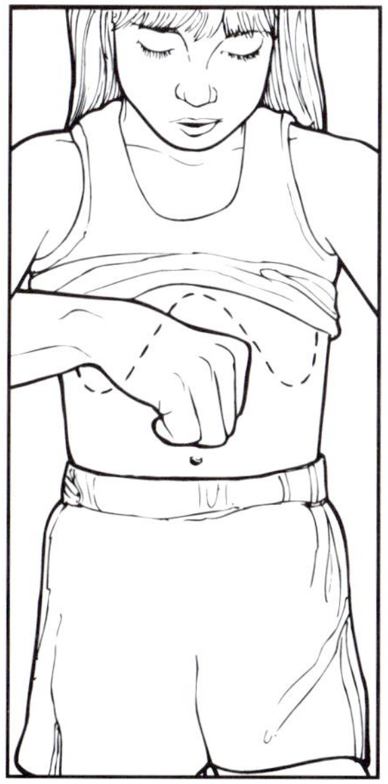

Figure 2

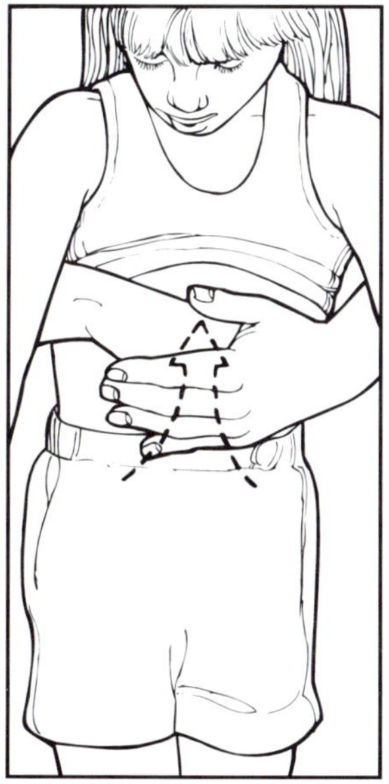

4. Support her body by bending the arm and leg nearest to you. (Figure 9)

c. If help has not yet been summoned, **call 911 or the rescue squad** now.

d. Return to the child and await medical assistance. Continue to observe her breathing. If breathing stops, proceed to Step 6.

Figure 9

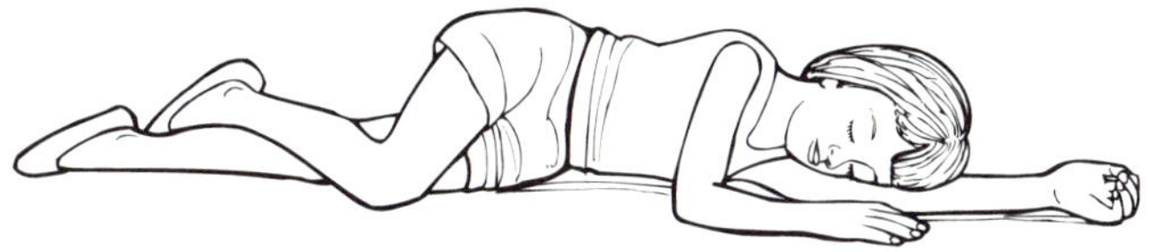

6. Give two rescue breaths.

a. Leaving your hand on the child's forehead, use your thumb and index finger to pinch her nose shut.

b. Place your mouth over the child's mouth, making a tight seal.

c. Give a breath for 1 to $1\frac{1}{2}$ seconds, pause, then give a second breath for 1 to $1\frac{1}{2}$ seconds. (Figure 10)

d. Look at or feel the child's chest when giving a breath—the chest should rise.

e. If the breath did not go in easily, reposition the child's head and try again.

Figure 10

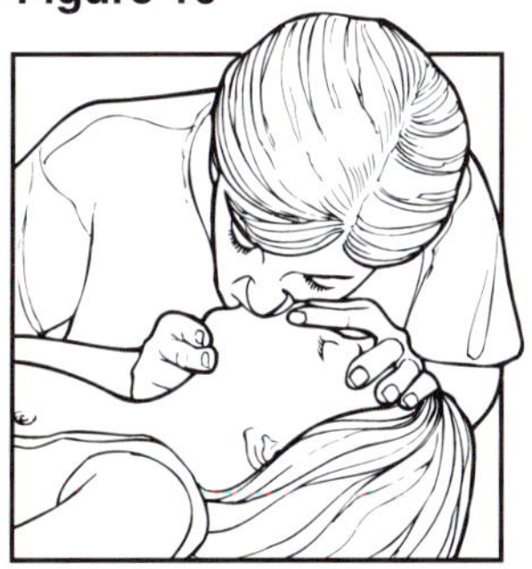

7. Determine if air is entering the child's lungs.

If air goes in easily and the child's chest rises, proceed with rescue breathing as instructed in **Rescue Breathing/Cardiopulmonary Resuscitation (CPR):** for children 1–8 years old, begin with Step 7, page 37; for children 8+ years, begin with Step 7, page 43.

If air does not go in easily and the child's chest does not rise, the airway remains blocked. Follow Steps 8–14.

d. If the child is not breathing, see **Rescue Breathing/ Cardiopulmonary Resuscitation (CPR):** for children 1–8 years old, begin with Step 6, page 35; for children 8+ years old, begin with Step 6, page 41. If the child is breathing, see **When to See a Doctor,** below.

When to See a Doctor

After the initial action is taken, take the child to see a doctor if any of the following apply:

- The child's windpipe is cleared of the foreign object and she begins to breathe on her own, but she had been unconscious.
- The child develops a fever and symptoms of a cold within a few days. (Part of the foreign object may have been inhaled into a lung, causing an infection.) Other symptoms to report include cough, fatigue, loss of appetite, and pain in the chest.
- The child has any difficulty breathing.

Home Treatment

Follow-up treatment involves observing the child over the next few days for the symptoms noted above.

nose shut; place your mouth over the child's mouth, making a tight seal. (Figure 5, 6)

2. Give a breath for 1 to $1\frac{1}{2}$ seconds, pause, then give a second breath for 1 to $1\frac{1}{2}$ seconds. You may have to deliver the breath with more force than usual, as water in the lungs may make it difficult for them to inflate.
3. Look at the child's chest when giving a breath—the chest should rise.
4. If the breath does not go in easily, reposition the child's head and try again.
5. If the breath still does not go in easily, see **Choking:** for infants, 0–1 year old, begin with Step 8, page 97; for children 1+ years old, begin with Step 8, page 109.

NOTE: *If a possibility of a back or neck injury exists, restrict treatment for choking to chest thrusts on infants and abdominal thrusts on children 1+ years old.*

Figure 5

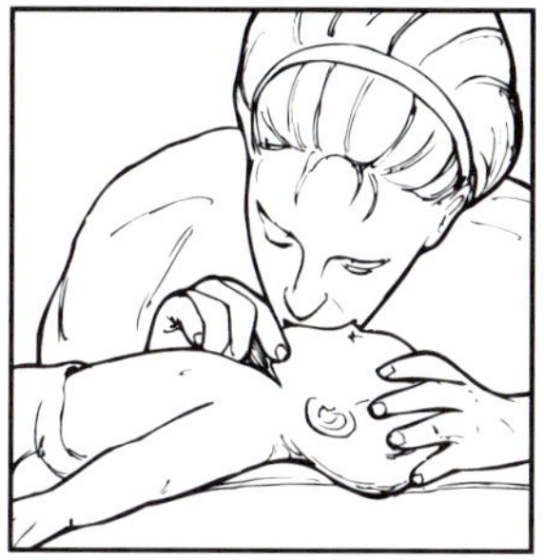

Figure 6

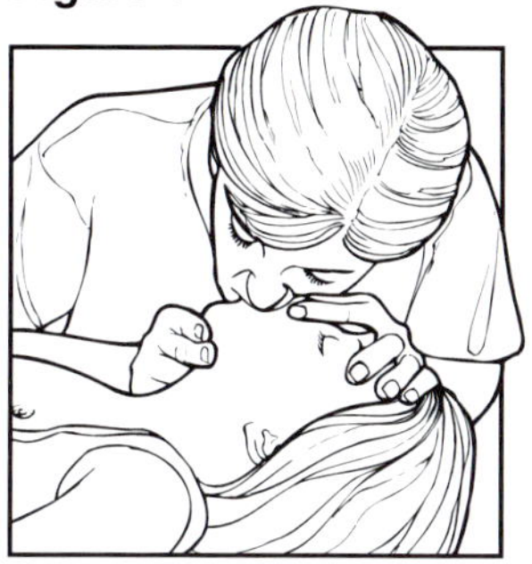

6. Check the child's pulse.

For an infant, 0–1 year, check the pulse in the upper arm. (Figure 7) For a child 1+ years, check the pulse on the side of the neck. (Figure 8) Check for 3–5 seconds. See **How to Check a Child's Vital Signs,** page 13, if necessary.

Figure 7

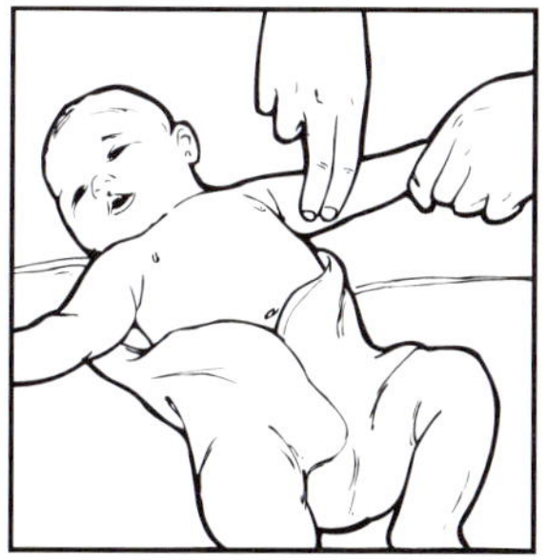

Figure 8

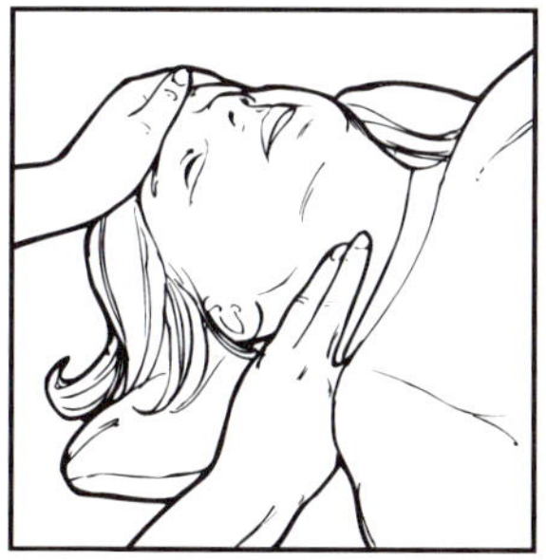

If a pulse is present,

a. Continue rescue breathing as you carefully transport the child out of the water:

- 0–8 years—one breath every 3 seconds
- 8+ years—one breath every 5 seconds

Do not bend or twist the child's body; keep her head in line with the rest of her body. If possible, use a board or some other flat surface to help transport the child.

2. Check for and treat the most life-threatening problems now.

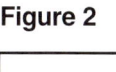

Check for signs of unconsciousness, no breathing, no pulse, bleeding, and shock. (Figure 2) See **Life-Threat Checklist,** page 23. **Call 911 or the rescue squad** as recommended in **Life-Threat Checklist.**

Once the most life-threatening problems have been attended to, you may proceed with further treatment as instructed below.

Figure 2

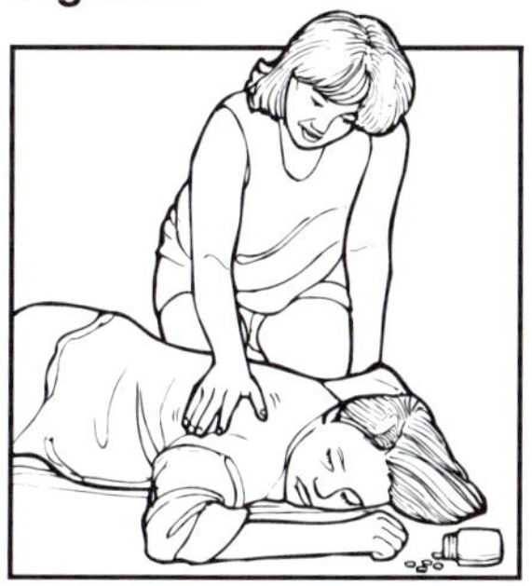

3. Check the child for signs of a drug overdose:

- Breathing—very slow, difficult, or absent (If there is no breathing, see **Rescue Breathing/Cardiopulmonary Resuscitation (CPR)** immediately: 0–1 year, page 27; 1–8 years, page 33; 8+ years, page 39.)
- Pulse—very rapid (0–8 years—more than 120 beats per minute; 8+ years—more than 100 beats per minute)
- Level of consciousness—drowsiness, difficulty in arousing from sleep, possible unconsciousness (If the child is unconscious, see **Rescue Breathing/ Cardiopulmonary Resuscitation (CPR)** immediately: 0–1 year, page 27; 1–8 years, page 33; 8+ years, page 39.)
- Absence of signs of traumatic injury that otherwise might have contributed to the child's condition (However, drug overdose is sometimes a suicide attempt, and there may be self-inflicted bruises, cuts, or other injuries.) (Figure 3)
- Combativeness, violence; uncooperativeness
- Extreme depression

Figure 3

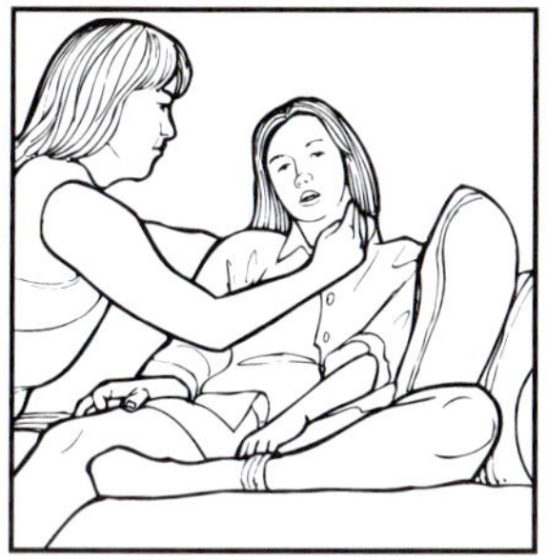

- The child has any fever and:
  - — is extremely irritable or much more tired or sleepy than usual.
  - — has difficulty breathing.
  - — has a stiff neck. (She cries loudly if you try to bend her head forward, she holds her neck straight, or she complains of pain in her neck.)
  - — is having a seizure.
  - — pulls her ear or complains of ear pain.
  - — develops a rash.
  - — will not eat.
  - — has not passed any urine for 12 hours.
  - — complains of pain when she passes urine or suddenly has to pass urine much more frequently than usual.
  - — complains of a sore throat.

Home Treatment

1. Take the child's temperature every 4 hours, around the clock, until it stabilizes between 98° and 99°F. Then take the temperature every 8 hours or when the child feels hot.
2. As long as fever continues, medicate the child with acetaminophen as directed on the product label and sponge-bathe her if instructed to do so by the doctor.
3. Give the child plenty of cool liquids.
4. Encourage the child to rest.
5. Report new signs of illness or an inability to reduce the fever to the doctor.

b. Take the child to the nearest hospital for injuries to other body parts.

7. Check the child and the injured area continuously.

a. Observe for shock; treat if necessary. See **Shock,** page 169.

b. Check an injured extremity for the presence of a pulse, blue or pale color, numbness, inability to wiggle toes or fingers, pain, and coldness. Loosen the splint if the injured area becomes increasingly swollen, if the limb becomes very blue or pale or cold, or if the child cannot feel your touch or wiggle his toes or fingers.

Splints and Slings

The joint above and the joint below a broken bone must be held still so that the bone does not move. For example, if the lower leg may be broken, the joints you must immobilize (hold still) are the knee and ankle. The instructions that follow call for the use of splints and slings to hold an injured part still. Move an injured extremity as little as possible when applying a splint or a sling.

Splints

A *splint* is a firm, long, straight object placed against an injured extremity to prevent the joint(s) from bending.

Items to Use for Splints

Piece of wood, broom, wooden spoon, umbrella, baseball bat, magazine or newspaper rolled tightly, pillow (for foot or toe), cane, pencil (for finger), branch (Figure 6)

Figure 6

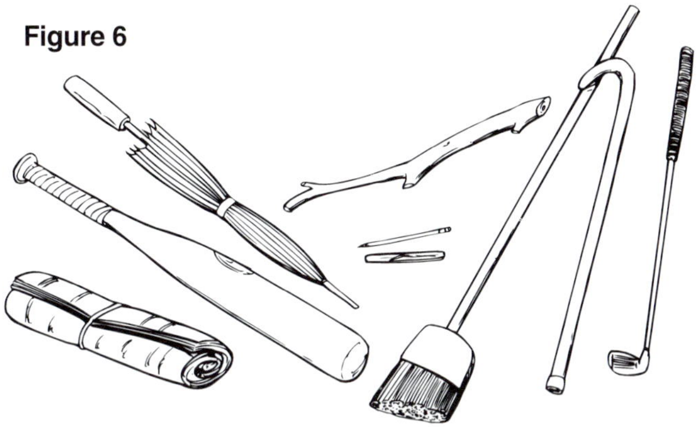

Straight Elbow

1. Place a pad (such as a small folded towel) in the child's armpit.
2. Place a padded splint along the underside of the child's arm, extending from the armpit to the hand.
3. Wrap the splint snugly with cloth. (Figure 19)

OR

1. Place a pad (such as a small folded towel) in the child's armpit.
2. Fold a pillow around the child's arm.
3. Wrap the pillow snugly with cloth or hold it in place with safety pins. (Figure 20)

Finger

Apply a padded splint along the underside of the child's finger. Wrap the splint snugly with cloth. (Figure 21)

Hip and Upper Leg

If you are unsure whether it is the hip or the pelvis that is broken, treat for pelvis. See **Pelvis,** page 137.

1. **Call 911 or the rescue squad** for transport to a medical facility.
2. While awaiting medical assistance, observe and treat for shock. (There may be a large amount of internal bleeding.) See **Shock,** page 169.
3. Do not allow the child to move his legs:
   - **a.** Place thick padding between the child's legs, along the entire length of the legs.
   - **b.** Tie the legs together with strips of cloth. Do this firmly enough to prevent movement. (Figure 22)

Figure 19

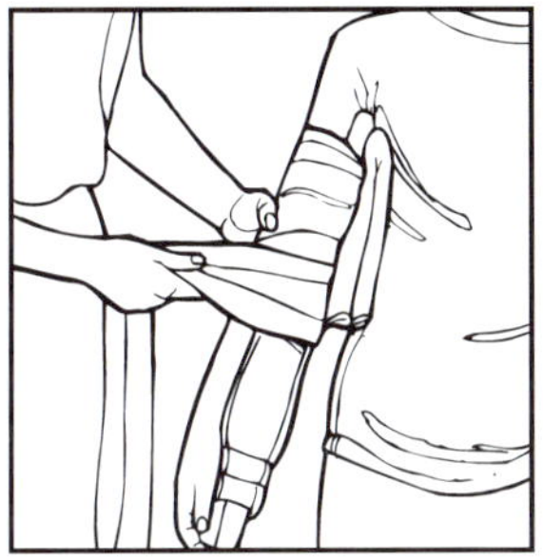

Figure 20

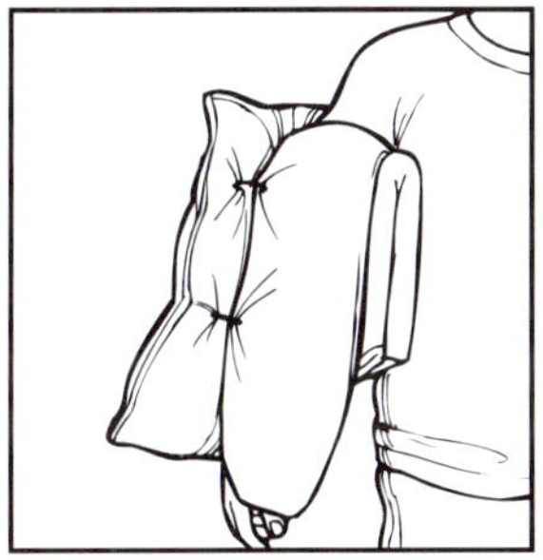

Figure 21

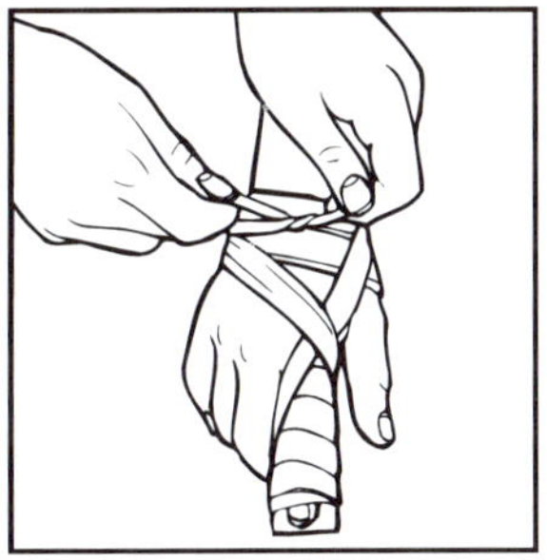

Figure 22

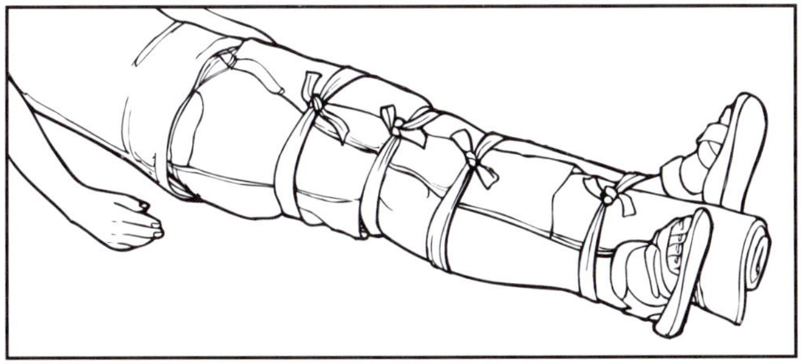

Ankle, Foot, or Toe

1. Remove the child's shoe gently, holding her foot and leg steady.
2. Place a pillow or a folded blanket under the calf—about one-third of the pillow or blanket should extend past the foot.
3. Fold the pillow or blanket around the calf and ankle. Wrap the pillow or blanket snugly with strips of cloth. (Figure 33)
4. Fold the rest of the pillow or blanket around the foot. You should be able to see the toes. Wrap the pillow or blanket snugly with strips of cloth. (Figure 34)
5. Raise the leg to decrease swelling.
6. Check the child's toes. If they are cold, pale or blue, or numb (the child cannot feel your touch), loosen the ties. Recheck every 15 minutes. (The ties will tighten as swelling increases.)
7. Apply ice, wrapped in plastic or cloth, to the injured area.

Figure 33

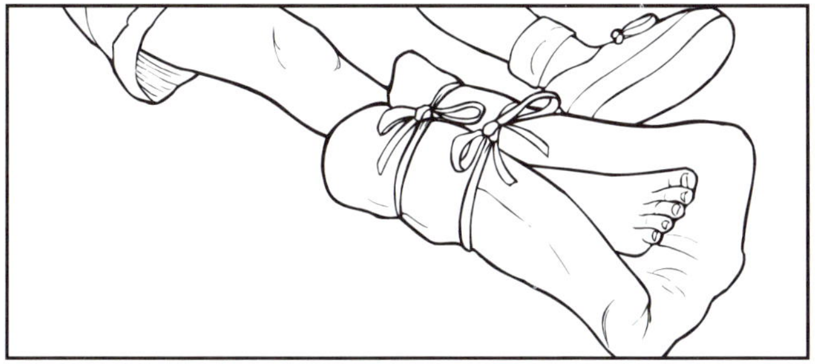

Figure 34

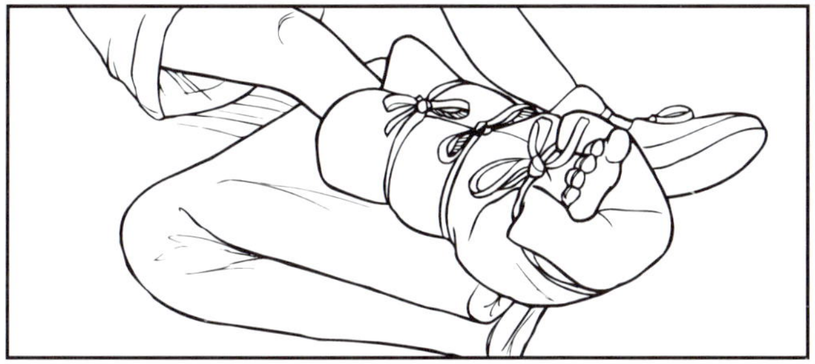

When to See a Doctor

Call 911 or rescue squad if previously instructed to do so. Otherwise, take the child to see a doctor if you think the child might have a fracture. Fractures and sprains have many of the same signs and may be correctly diagnosed only by X rays. If the injured body part was twisted or received a forceful blow and is cold, blue or pale, or numb; is unable to bear weight or move; is crooked or deformed; has a bone sticking out through the skin; or is painful, swollen, and bruised, call the child's doctor. Bandage any wound and splint a suspected fracture as recommended in the preceding pages before bringing the child to a medical facility.

Immediate Action

1. Look at the surroundings and the general appearance of the child.

(Take a few seconds.)

- Was the child's head hit forcibly by a sharp or blunt object?
- Was there a severe fall (perhaps from a tree, from playground equipment, or out of a window)? (Figure 1)
- Was the child thrown from a motor vehicle or bicycle?
- If the child is an infant, was he shaken vigorously?

If the answer to any of the above is *yes,* there could be a severe head injury.

Figure 1

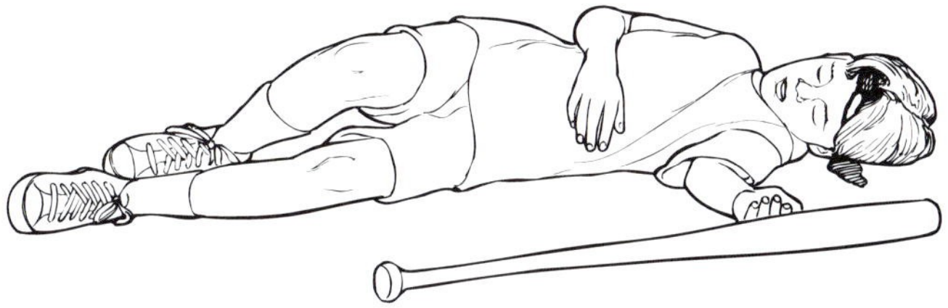

2. Check for and treat most life-threatening problems now.

Check for signs of unconsciousness, no breathing, no pulse, bleeding, and shock. (Figure 2) See **Life-Threat Checklist,** page 23. **Call 911 or the rescue squad** as recommended in **Life-Threat Checklist.**

NOTE: *If the child is unconscious, assume there is a back or neck injury. Handle the child carefully. Do not bend or twist his body or neck. If there is bleeding, press only lightly on the wound, in case the skull is broken. Put a bandage in place when bleeding is controlled.*

Figure 2

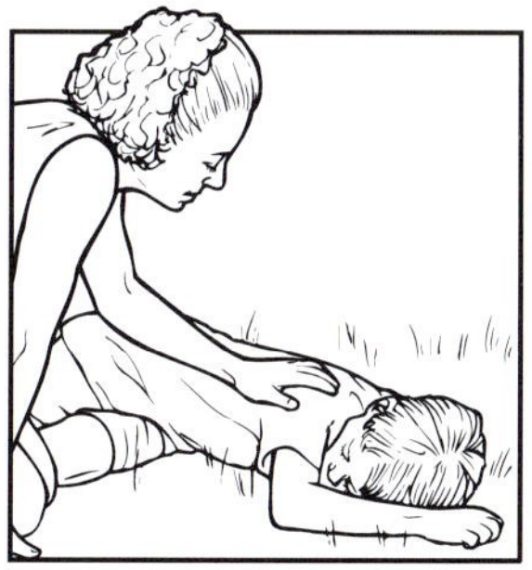

Once the most life-threatening problems have been attended to, you may proceed with further treatment as instructed below.

- If the child is unconscious, follow the instructions on pages 145–147, **If the Child Is Unconscious (Not Responsive).**
- If the child is conscious but the injury is serious, follow the instructions on pages 147–149, **If the**

- Gastrointestinal signs
  The child is nauseated and/or vomiting.
- Other
  The child has a headache, is crying, and/or is irritable. (Young children may be in pain but may not be able to tell you where they hurt.)

If none of the above signs are present and only a minor bruise or head wound is present, refer to **When to See a Doctor** and **Home Treatment,** page 150. Otherwise, proceed with instructions as follows.

2. Seek medical assistance.

a. **Call 911 or the rescue squad** if:
   - The child is having difficulty breathing.
   - The child cannot move one or more body parts.
   - The child has a very slow pulse (0–1 year—less than 80 beats per minute; 1+ years—less than 60 beats per minute).
   - The child is bleeding uncontrollably.
   - The child is having seizures.
   - The child becomes unconscious.

   Proceed to Step 3.

b. Call the child's doctor if:
   - Clear fluid or blood is draining from the ears, nose, and/or mouth.
   - The child is confused.
   - The child cannot answer simple age-appropriate questions.
   - The child has black eyes or blackness behind the ears.
   - The child is drowsy, has blurred vision, nausea, or is vomiting.

   Follow the doctor's recommendations; the child may have to be examined by a physician.

e. If there is no vomiting within the *next* 30 minutes, do not repeat. Tickle the back of the child's throat with your finger to stimulate vomiting. Remember to have the child vomit into a bucket or bowl so you can take a sample to the medical facility.

f. Give the child one or two glasses of water or milk to dilute the poison.

g. Once the child has vomited, bring the child, the poison container, and a sample of the vomit to the medical facility.

7. If you cannot reach medical assistance by telephone,

a. Dilute the poison—if the child is awake and alert, give him one or two glasses of milk or water.

b. Observe and treat for symptoms of breathing difficulty. See **Breathing Difficulty—General,** page 71. If the child stops breathing, see **Rescue Breathing/Cardiopulmonary Resuscitation (CPR):** 0–1 year, page 27; 1–8 years, page 33; 8+ years, page 39.

c. Treat for shock. See **Shock,** page 169.

d. Transport the child to the nearest medical facility.

2. Check for and treat the most life-threatening problems now.

Call 911 or the rescue squad if any of the following applies:

- The child fell onto a stationary object that pierced through a part of her body (impaled her) and she cannot be moved. (Figure 2)
- The object has gone through the chest, abdomen, or skull.
- Bleeding is severe, with large amounts of blood.

Check for signs of unconsciousness, no breathing, no pulse, bleeding, and shock. (Figure 3) See **Life-Threat Checklist,** page 23. **Call 911 or the rescue squad** as recommended in **Life-Threat Checklist,** if you have not already done so.

Once the most life-threatening problems have been attended to, you may proceed with further treatment as instructed below.

3. Control the bleeding.

a. Do not move or remove the object.

b. Apply direct pressure to the area *around* the point of bleeding. Do not put pressure on the object itself. (Figure 4)

c. If bleeding does not slow down in 5 minutes, press more firmly.

d. If bleeding does not slow down in 5 more minutes, apply pressure to the nearest appropriate pressure point. (See **If Bleeding Cannot be Immediately Controlled,** pages 66–68.)

Figure 2

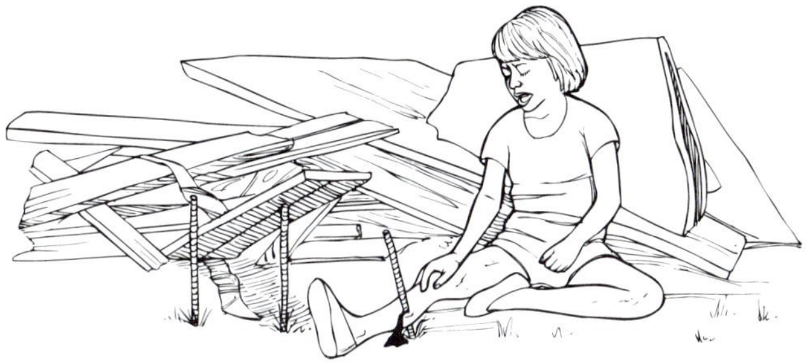

Figure 3

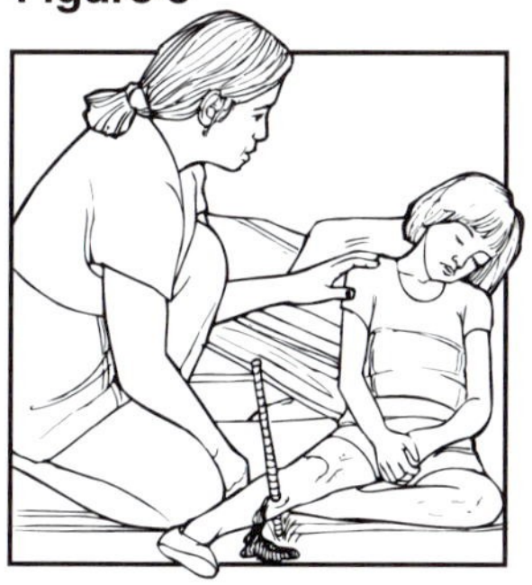

Figure 4

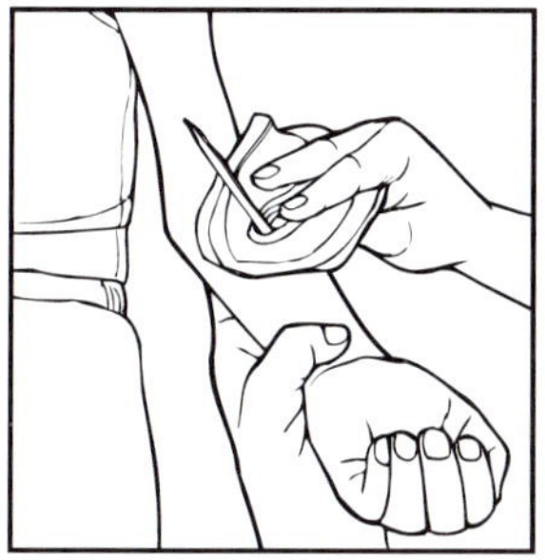

8. Reduce the child's fever, if present.

See **Fever,** page 125.

When to See a Doctor

Take the child to see a doctor if either of the following applies:

- The child had a seizure and has not been diagnosed or treated for a seizure disorder before.
- You are instructed to do so by the doctor.

Home Treatment

Once the child returns home from the medical facility, do the following:

1. Maintain the child's temperature below 101°F, or as instructed by the child's doctor. See **Fever,** page 125.
2. Report an inability to reduce the fever or any recurrence of the seizure to the doctor.

and neck, keeping them in line with the body. Do not move the head independently of the body. See ***Back and Neck Injuries,*** *page 45, for positioning techniques.*

Position the child on her side if:

- the child is unconscious, breathing, and you do not suspect a head, back, or neck injury.
- there is heavy bleeding from the jaw or lower face.
- the child is vomiting.

Place the child in the recovery position:

a. Kneel beside the child.

b. Turn the child onto her side by pulling her toward you.

c. For infants 0–1 year, hold the infant in position or support the infant's body by placing rolled-up clothing or a small blanket along her torso.

d. For children 1+ years, hold the child in position or support the child's body by bending the arm and leg nearest to you. (Figure 3)

e. Position the child's head to keep the airway open. The head should not be bent toward the chest.

Figure 3

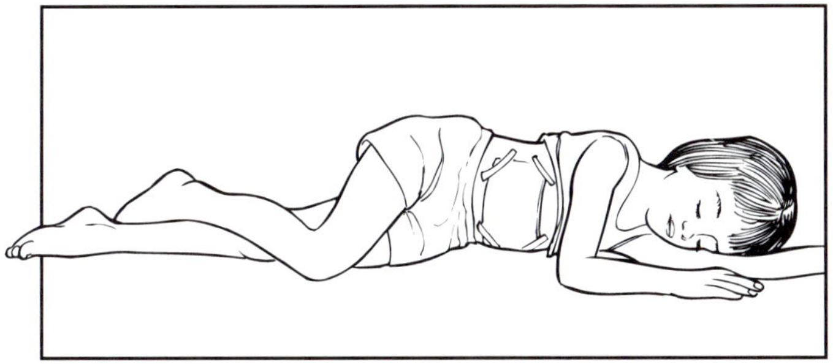

Position the child on her back if:

- the child is conscious.
- there is no vomiting or bleeding from the mouth.
- the child is unconscious and not breathing.

6. Position the child's legs.

Raise the child's legs 8–12 inches if:

- you do not suspect a leg or pelvic fracture.
- you do not suspect a back or neck injury.
- moving the child's legs does not cause pain.

Use a pillow, a blanket, or clothing to support the

Figure 4

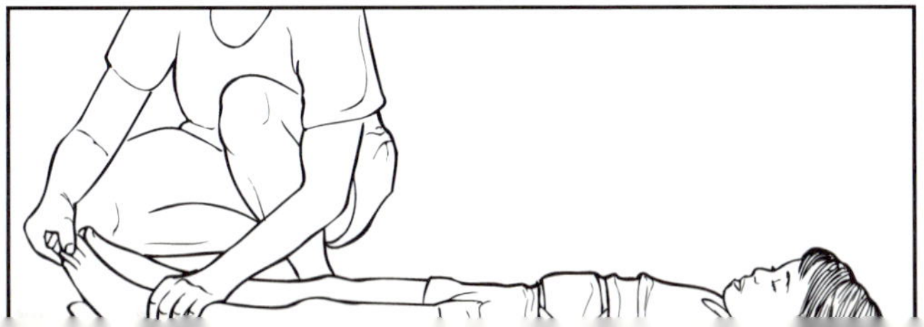

Coping Strategies

Ask the hospital staff if you can be with the infant during medical procedures. If this is not possible, remain nearby to comfort the child after procedures. If the infant must be admitted to the hospital, at least one parent should try to be with the infant as much as possible. Many hospitals have sleeping accommodations for a parent in the infant's room, excluding intensive-care units. If the infant's condition allows, a parent may be able to perform routine care, such as bathing, feeding, and rocking.

Provide the infant with stimulation in the hospital. If allowed by the hospital staff, hang a familiar mobile above the crib, place musical toys in the crib, or place stuffed animals by the infant's head. Leaving an article of clothing or a handkerchief near the infant's head will make him feel your presence by your scent.

The infant may want a parent or caregiver near him at all times for several days after discharge from the hospital. Plan to spend extra time with the infant to allow him to feel secure again.

Toddlers (1–3 Years)

Stressors	Behavioral reactions
Separation	Protest: The toddler cries for the parent or caregiver, verbally attacks others, engages in physical fighting (kicking, biting, hitting), tries to escape to find the parent or caregiver, clings to the parent or caregiver and physically tries to force him or her to stay, and cries inconsolably. Despair: Later, the child may show despair by becoming passive, depressed, and uninterested in her environment; by refusing to talk; and by losing newly learned skills. The child may be angry with the parent or caregiver for leaving her and may refuse to cooperate with him or her.

injured as punishment for something he did wrong. He then has to cope with feelings of guilt, shame, and fear. The child may become withdrawn. Because he may feel that he has let his parents down, he may become very quiet in the presence of the parents and/or may demonstrate extremely obedient behavior to win back the parents' approval. The child may also fantasize that a medical procedure will be much worse than it actually is and may fear a hospital staff member wearing a mask and gloves because he or she looks like an imagined monster.

Bodily injury and pain	The preschooler is able to associate past events with present ones and expects the same results to occur. If the last medicine the nurse gave him tasted awful, he will expect the next dose of medicine to taste awful, and he will verbally and physically resist its administration. The preschooler has a limited understanding of his body and how it functions. He views intrusive procedures such as injections, intravenous therapy, and blood sampling as attacks on his body. He does not understand that a hole made in his skin will seal itself and therefore fears that all his blood and "insides" will leak out. A bandage will help calm such fears. Because a preschooler fears mutilation, he thinks that surgery performed on any body part will result in the loss of that body part. Without preparation for a medical procedure, the child will imagine an event that is much worse than what is really going to happen and therefore will physically and verbally resist approach by a hospital staff member. Even with preparation, many children will resist procedures, but not as aggressively or for as long as if they had not been prepared. With preparation they also will settle down more quickly after the procedure is completed. Between the ages of 4 and 5, many preschoolers begin to show an increased level of self-control when feeling pain. Children of this age are also aware of cultural expectations such as "big kids don't cry," and may try to

child whether he will have bandages or a cast. Bandaging a doll exactly as the child will be bandaged is very helpful in preparing the child for planned procedures.

Inform the child's nurse when you know or suspect that the child is experiencing pain. Children may not admit they feel pain, sometimes because they fear they will receive an injection. Most pain medications are given intravenously or by mouth, so reassure the child that the medicine will hurt only a bit or not at all, and that it will help him feel better. Nurses often rely on parents to interpret nonverbal cues indicating that the child needs something, especially with a child who is quiet, shy, or attempting to be brave.

You can also relieve the child's pain by helping him relax through the use of deep breathing. Show the child how to inhale a deep breath of air through his nose, hold it for 2 seconds, and then blow it out slowly and completely through pursed lips, as if blowing out birthday candles. Repeat this several times. Deep breathing helps muscles relax, which can help relieve even significant pain. In addition, focusing the child's attention on breathing rather than on the pain helps him cope with it better. For this reason, distraction through such activities as playing a game, coloring or drawing, working with clay, or watching television is also helpful.

School-Age Children (6–12 Years)

Stressors	Behavioral reactions
Separation	Protest and despair are not usually typical of a school-age child, as the child is increasingly able to cope with separation. The youngest child may still require a parent's presence, however, as the stress of hospitalization causes her to regress to an earlier, preschool level of development. The older school-age child often reacts more to separation from her peers and her usual activities than to

may threaten her sense of security. The child will still expect some degree of discipline and structure from her parents. This, when balanced by compassion, support, and physical assistance as needed, will aid the child in coping with the crisis.

Prepare the child for medical procedures, treatments, diagnostic tests, or surgery with honest explanations in terms the child can understand. Avoid details that may only add to her confusion and fear. Ask the child's nurses, doctors, or therapists to assist you with explanations. Use pictures or examples of related experiences to aid the child's understanding. Younger children may benefit from handling bandages; a surgical mask, cap, and gown; or medical equipment, as allowed. To determine her degree of understanding and to clarify misunderstandings she may have about her treatment, ask the child to describe to you the procedures that are being performed. Address the child's nurses, doctors, and therapists by name and explain their roles, to help her perceive them as familiar people rather than as strangers intent on hurting her.

Allow the child to perform as much care by herself as her condition allows. Provide crafts or workbooks to enhance a feeling of productivity and accomplishment.

Encourage visitation by other family members and friends as appropriate and allowed by hospital policy. Keep the child informed about family activities and reassure her that she is missed at home.

If the child is going to be physically disabled or disfigured, whether temporarily or permanently, she is going to require a great deal of emotional support. This is especially true for children of 11 or 12 years, because of their deeper understanding of the limitations imposed by a disability and their more developed sense of time. Concern with body image also becomes increasingly important as the child approaches adolescence, making evaluated in the context of other symptoms and other stressful situations, such as problems he is having at school, at home, or with his peer group.

Coping Strategies

Encourage visits, letters, or phone calls from the child's peers to reassure him that they have not forgotten him. It is important, however, to limit the child's social time so that he is not deprived of the rest he needs to recover.

The adolescent usually will not welcome the constant presence of parents or other family members at his bedside. Because the adolescent perceives himself to be more like an adult than a child, he believes he is capable of making decisions for himself and feels he does not need constant parental protection. It is important to provide the child with periods of privacy at the hospital, not only to help him learn to assert himself in a new environment, but also to convey to him your belief that he is capable of managing many of his needs independently.

Encourage the child to talk about his feelings of loneliness and isolation. Reassure him that physical separation from family and friends does not mean they have forgotten about him.

It is important to help the child regain a sense of control as soon as possible. Allow him to make choices about his care or daily activities, as his condition permits. Time not allotted to treatments, diagnostic tests, examinations by hospital staff, or other scheduled hospital procedures should be time when the child can engage in social activities, do schoolwork, or rest, and should be scheduled by the child. Reinforce the idea that all his needs must be met at some time during the day but that he can decide when.

Prepare the child for procedures, treatments, diagnostic tests, or surgery with honest explanations, in terms the child can understand. Clarify any misunderstandings to the best of your ability. Relay the child's fears to his

INTRODUCTION

This first-aid guide has been designed for use by parents, grandparents, childcare providers, and other members of the nonmedical public who at some time are responsible for the care of a child 0–18 years of age. Of course, conscientious attempts to prevent injury should be the caregiver's top priority. Nonetheless, accidents can happen, and illnesses sometimes occur with little warning. As the child's caregiver, you may be the first to respond when an injury has occurred or during a critical stage of illness. Therefore, it is important that you know what to do in those important first few minutes, either to prevent the child from becoming more seriously injured or to improve the child's condition.

The topics addressed in this guide include those life-threatening injuries or complications of illness that occur most frequently in children. They are the types of injuries or complications that require sound attention within minutes of their occurrence.

In this guide, the discussion of each topic includes instructions to call 911 or a rescue squad to summon emergency medical help if certain life-threatening signs exist. It is often much safer to have professional help come to the child than for you to drive the child to a medical facility and risk having the child's condition become critically worse in the car.

A child's body has the ability to recover from injury or illness more quickly than that of an adult, but it can also become critically ill much more quickly—and unpredictably. Partly for this reason, it is important that you know how to attend to life-threatening problems before professional help arrives. Although in many communities professional help can respond to an emergency within 5 minutes of a phone call, a child can begin to suffer brain damage after only 4 minutes of lack of oxygen due to a cessation in breathing, severe blood or fluid loss, heart failure, or shock. A child with a broken neck or other fracture, if not immediately attended to, may move in such a way as to complicate the injury further. It has been shown that in a life-threatening situation, a combination of prompt first-respondent care and care given by medical professionals dramatically increases the chances of a favorable recovery.

Many people doubt that they could provide effective emergency care for a child. This is usually because they are not sure what they are supposed to, or can, do. This guide provides you with the information you need not only to know when a child's injury or illness is serious, but also to know what to do first, what *not* to do, when to call for emergency medical help, and when a child should be seen by a doctor.

The guide is not intended to serve as a substitute for classroom instruction in first aid, but rather as an aid to such instruction, with which you will have the opportunity to practice performing the recommended procedures. The most effective way of learning anything is by doing it, which is why it is extremely important to learn and practice lifesaving skills such as rescue breathing, cardiopulmonary resuscitation (CPR), and choking intervention in a supervised setting. Your confidence in your ability to respond effectively to a childhood emergency should increase after having been provided with first-aid information and the opportunity to apply it in practice sessions.

Format

The bulk of this guide consists of first-aid information for various situations, arranged in alphabetical order in Part III for ease of reference. Part II, **Critical Care,** deals with rescue breathing and cardiopulmonary resuscitation (CPR), and occurs before the other first-aid sections due to its importance. Because rescue breathing/CPR techniques differ for victims of different ages, this section is divided into three subsections covering care given to infants 0–1 year, small children 1–8 years, and older children 8+ years. These instructions are consistent with the standards set by the American Heart Association.

Following the section on rescue breathing/CPR, each chapter in Part III begins with **Safety Highlights.** This provides important dos and don'ts of safe care at a glance.

Immediate Action follows next, with step-by-step instructions for assessing the emergency and giving care. The steps are listed in descending order of priority, from the child's most immediate to least immediate needs. The first course of action is always to observe the child and the surroundings to gather clues about what happened and what the injury might be. The purpose of doing this is twofold: to stop yourself from automatically moving an injured child and possibly causing more harm in the event of a fracture or back or neck injury, and to help yourself accurately assess how seriously ill or injured the child is and what his or her needs are.

Next, check for and attend to any life-threatening problems before doing anything else. In this step, you should refer to the **Life-Threat Checklist,** a reference flow chart located in Part II, page 23. This flow chart was created to help you quickly identify the child's most important life-threatening problems first, regardless of the type of injury or illness. At appropriate points in the checklist, you are advised to call for emergency medical help and referred to the sections on rescue breathing and CPR, if these procedures are called for. Once the child's most life-threatening problems have been attended to, you should begin attending to the specific injury or illness. This prioritizing of needs and first-aid steps is consistent with standards set by the American Red Cross.

Following Immediate Action, **When to See a Doctor** provides information to help you decide whether or not the child requires professional medical attention. However, the child's own doctor may be able to provide you with recommendations for contacting him or her, and it is usually best to follow those recommendations.

Home Treatment is included in each first-aid section to provide you with information about follow-up care and about how to treat an injury or complication of illness that is not severe enough to require professional medical attention. Signs and symptoms to watch for are included.

In addition to the first-aid sections for specific situations, the guide includes various reference sections. The following reference sections are in Part I at the front of the guide.

First-Aid Supplies to Have on Hand assists you in preparing for a medical emergency. Items on the supply list are among those most commonly used in first-aid situations.

How to Get Emergency Medical Help tells you how to access the emergency medical system and details the information that you or another caller will have to relay to an operator. Because some communities do not have the 911 emergency phone system, space is provided for filling in the phone number of your local rescue squad.

Emergency Phone Numbers provides space for you to write the numbers of significant individuals or organizations who may need to be contacted in an emergency, such as the Poison Control Center.

Care of an Injured Child Within a Group gives tips for dealing with and attending to the other children if an injury or illness occurs in a group setting.

How to Check a Child's Vital Signs details the methods of assessing a child's pulse rate and character, breathing rate and pattern, and temperature. This information will be important to medical professionals in diagnosing the problem and determining the child's most immediate needs.

At the back of the guide is a section entitled **Meeting the Child's Emotional Needs.** This section is not intended to be read in an emergency. Instead, it provides information for the emotional care of an ill or injured child after the crisis has passed. Children can be negatively affected by the stress of a medical emergency and hospitalization. This section will make you aware of the types of behavior to expect in children of different ages and assist you in helping the child cope with the stressful event. Following the section on emotional needs is a list of references for further reading.

Throughout the guide, an effort has been made to keep cross-referencing to a minimum and to provide you with the information you need to care for an injury or illness in the pages devoted to that particular topic. However, many medical problems overlap. For example, a child with a head injury may also have a back or neck injury, making a reference to that topic necessary.

To aid understanding, the instructions in this guide are quite detailed. If you wait until an emergency occurs to read the instructions, you will waste valuable time. It is best to read and practice the various instructions before an emergency occurs. Then you should be able to perform emergency assessments and procedures by referring to the key steps in large, bold print.

You will note that the guide alternates in its references to a child's gender, sometimes using *he/him/his* and other times using *she/her/hers.* This is done not to make instructions gender-specific; rather, all first-aid instructions apply to both sexes, regardless of which pronouns are used.

Finally, you are to be commended for taking the time and initiative to become better prepared to care for a child in a medical emergency. Childcare is a serious responsibility, and the more knowledgeable you are, the better equipped you will be to face its challenges.

- Adhesive strip bandages of different sizes (for example, Band-Aid® Brand Adhesive Bandages)
- Sterile gauze pads of different sizes
- Sterile nonadherent pads of different sizes
- Rolls of gauze bandage, $\frac{1}{2}$ inch and 3 inches wide (to hold pads in place)
- Elastic bandage (for sprains)
- Adhesive tape, paper and cloth, 1 inch wide
- Triangular bandage with safety pins (for a sling)
- Cotton balls
- Cotton-tipped swabs
- Calamine lotion
- Thermometers, rectal and oral
- Petroleum jelly (for rectal thermometers)
- Scissors
- Syrup of ipecac (to stimulate vomiting of poison or drug)
- Children's nonaspirin fever reducer (available in drops for infants, liquid and tablets for children; also stock in rectal suppository form)
- Antibiotic ointment (to be used on advice from a doctor)
- Hydrogen peroxide (for cleaning wounds)
- Ice pack (available in commercial form)
- Aspirator or bulb syringe
- Insect-sting kit (for children with severe allergic reactions to insect stings; must be prescribed by a doctor)

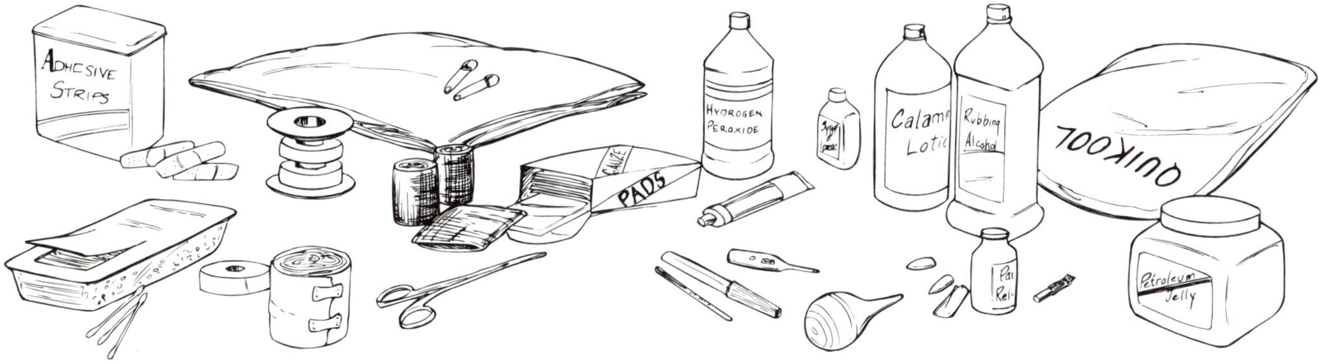

1. **Call 911 or the rescue squad.**
   #______________________________________

   If you do not have 911 service or a rescue squad is not available, call the operator by dialing "0."
2. Give the operator your name and the location of the emergency.
3. Give the operator the phone number of the telephone you are using.
4. Describe what happened and to how many children.
5. Describe the child's general appearance (not responding, not breathing, and so on).
6. Describe what is being done for the child.
7. Listen for instructions.
8. Hang up only when told to do so by the operator.

Rescue Squad

#__________________________________

Poison Control Center

#__________________________________

Local Hospital

Name______________________________

#__________________________________

Child's Doctor

Name______________________________

Office #____________________________

Emergency #________________________

Other Doctors

Name______________________________

Specialty___________________________

Office #____________________________

Emergency #________________________

Name______________________________

Specialty___________________________

Office #____________________________

Emergency #________________________

Family Members

Name______________________________

Home #____________________________

Work #____________________________

Name______________________________

Home #____________________________

Work #____________________________

Neighbors

Name______________________________

Home #____________________________

Work #____________________________

Name______________________________

Home #____________________________

Work #____________________________

If a child is injured in a group setting, such as a classroom, a day-care center, or a Scouting or sporting event, attention will have to be paid to the other children as well as the injured child. It is a stressful experience for children to witness injury or illness, especially in someone of similar age. Some children may openly express this stress as fear and panic, with screaming, crying, and vocal insistence that you, the care provider, "do something." Other children may withdraw, unable to speak.

In any case, the reactions of the children may require attention, and yet your first concern must be the injured or ill child. Thus, if at all possible, you must have someone else attend to the needs of the other children. If no other adult who can help is with you, follow these steps:

1. If adults are in the area, shout to them for help. Otherwise, phone someone. If you cannot leave the injured or ill child to make a phone call, direct one of the other children, if developmentally able, to call. Write down the phone number for the child, including 911 if necessary.
2. Act as calmly as possible. Tell the other children that the injured or ill child is being cared for and that you must pay attention to him right now. Let them know that someone is coming to help and will take care of their needs too.
3. When an adult arrives, direct her to lead the other children away from the scene, out of view. (If there is no possibility of adult assistance, choose a developmentally able, capable child from the group to do this.) The assistant should distract the children with an activity if possible, but continue to check with you periodically about the child's condition and provide reports to the group. (If available, a second assistant may do this.)

   Children's thoughts will still be focused on their friend, regardless of diversionary activity, and their imaginations may create a situation that is much worse than the reality. Thus, it is better to keep them informed of events than to disregard their fears and pretend that nothing is happening. When providing information to the children, the assistant should keep details to a minimum and avoid predicting the child's outcome. Instead, the assistant should reassure the children that doctors and nurses will try to help their friend feel better.
4. Do not attempt to transport all the children to the medical facility if you must accompany the injured or ill child. An assistant should stay with the children.

It is not uncommon for children who have witnessed an emergency to relate the situation to themselves. If a child's friend broke her leg, she too may start to limp, complain of pain, and insist that her leg is broken. This reaction may be expressed immediately or days, even weeks, later. The child needs validation that she is, indeed, okay. This will strengthen her feeling of security and diminish her fears. You can help this child by allowing her to verbalize her feelings, providing truthful answers to her questions, correcting her misconceptions, and engaging in activity that demonstrates that she is well. Share these concerns with the child's parent or guardian, if possible, and encourage them to attend to the child's needs.

Checking a Pulse

One way of telling how fast the heart is beating is by taking the pulse. Each time the heart beats, it sends blood into the arteries, causing them to stretch. You can feel this stretching as a pulsation, or throb, in many arteries all over the body. However, it will be felt more strongly or found more readily in some arteries more than others, the best locations of which differ between children and adults. The most appropriate locations for taking the pulse of both infants and older children are provided here.

To Take the Pulse

1. If the child is crying or anxious, calm her or distract her with a toy.
2. Using the tips of your first two fingers, find the correct location of the pulse as described below. (Do not use your thumb, because it has its own pulse that may be mistaken for the child's pulse.)

   Infants 0–1 Year

   Place your first two fingers inside the infant's upper arm, about halfway between the armpit and the elbow. (Figure 1)

   Children 1+ Years

   Place your first two fingers in the middle of the child's neck, over the Adam's apple (the firm, bulging area). Slide your fingers toward you into the groove on the side of the neck, below the angle of the jaw. (Figure 2)

Range of Normal Heart Rates at Rest

Age	Beats per minute
0–1 month	100–170
1 month–1 year	100–140
1–3 years	100–130
3–8 years	80–100
8+ years	60–90

The heart rate will be **higher** with activity, crying, fever, dehydration, shock, anxiety, hot environmental temperature, or breathing difficulty.

The heart rate will be **lower** with some illnesses or injuries, such as head injuries, deep sleep, or cold environmental temperature.

Figure 1

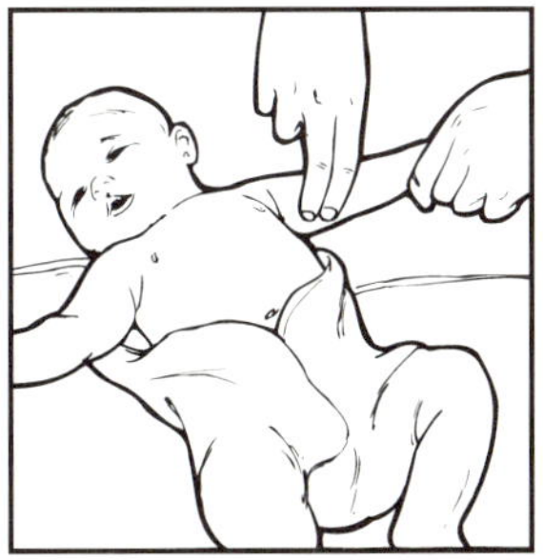

Figure 2

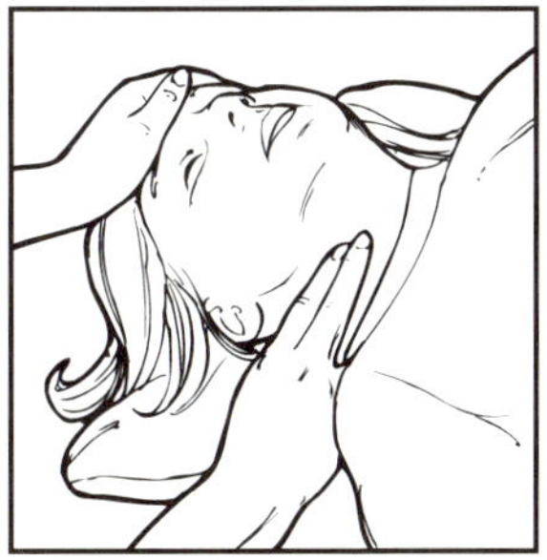

VITAL SIGNS

3. Press down gently.
4. If you do not feel the pulse after 2–3 seconds, move your fingers slightly to find the correct location. Press gently again. Repeat again, if necessary, allowing a full 5–10 seconds to determine whether or not there is a pulse. Do not rush—a weak pulse may be hard to feel.
5. Count the number of throbs (heartbeats) in 1 minute, and compare it to the **Range of Normal Heart Rates at Rest,** as given on page 13.
6. Note whether the pulse feels strong or weak.
7. If there is no pulse, see **Rescue Breathing/ Cardiopulmonary Resuscitation (CPR):** 0–1 year, page 27; 1–8 years, page 33; 8+ years, page 39.

Checking Respiration (Breathing)

Children generally breathe faster than adults do, especially when they are active. Infants use their stomach muscles to breathe, rather than expanding their chests as adults do, so it is important to look at the infant's abdomen as well as her chest when checking for breathing problems. An infant's breathing pattern is usually irregular—she may breathe rapidly for a few seconds, stop for a few seconds, breathe in a slower and easier pattern for a while, and then repeat the cycle.

To Count the Breathing Rate

1. Count when the child is at rest or asleep, if possible. If she is awake, distract the child with a toy or hold the child to calm her, if necessary.
2. While you watch the child's chest or abdomen, count how many times the child breathes in 1 full minute. If necessary, lightly place your hand on the chest or abdomen to assist with counting.
3. If you are not sure if the child is breathing, place your face near the child's nose and mouth. Listen and feel for air movement from the mouth or nose while also watching the chest and abdomen.
4. Look for signs of breathing difficulty. A child experiencing breathing difficulty might be
   - Breathing much more rapidly than usual (0–1 year—more than sixty times per minute; 1+ years—more than forty times per minute).
   - Pulling in her chest and/or stomach muscles so deeply that you can see her ribs much more easily than usual.
   - Looking very anxious, with trouble breathing, or telling you she is having trouble breathing.
   - Having difficulty swallowing, which is causing drooling, and breathing with her mouth wide open and her chin jutting forward.
   - Breathing noisily.
   - Experiencing hoarseness with a cough that sounds like a barking seal.
   - Experiencing a congested cough, and there is a "rattling" sensation when you feel her chest or back.
   - Gasping for air.
   - Wheezing, or making whistling noises as she breathes in and/or out.

Range of Normal Breathing Rates at Rest

Age	Breaths per minute
0–1 month	40–60
1 month–1 year	30–40
1–3 years	20–30
3–8 years	20–25
8+ years	16–20

The breathing rate will be **higher** with anxiety, difficulty with breathing (such as asthma), allergic reaction, fever, high blood sugar (as with diabetes), respiratory infection, or rigorous activity.

The breathing rate will be **lower** with shock, drug overdose or poisoning, deep sleep, or severe head injury.

To Take the Temperature

Oral Method

1. Use an oral thermometer. (The type will be labeled on the package. Many oral thermometers have a blue color at the flat end. The silver-tipped end is long and narrow.) (Figure 3)
2. "Shake down" the thermometer so that the mercury (interior silver-colored line) is no higher than 94°F.
3. Wait at least 10 minutes after the child has had anything to eat or drink.
4. Place the silver-tipped end of the thermometer under the child's tongue.
5. Have the child close her mouth completely. Stay with the child to be sure she keeps her mouth closed. (Figure 4)
6. Remove the thermometer after 5 minutes.

Figure 3

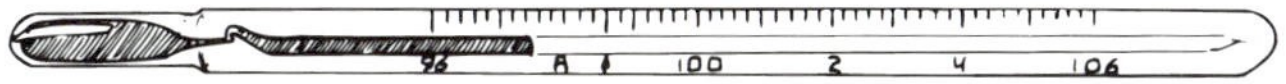

oral thermometer

Figure 4

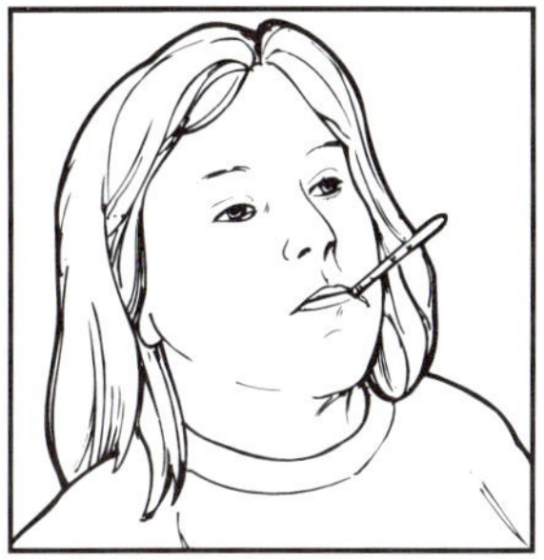

Measuring Method: Oral

When to Use

- Child is over 3 years old.
- Child is alert and awake.
- Child is cooperative and dependable (will not bite down on thermometer).

When Not to Use

- Child is unconscious.
- Child has mouth sores or injury.
- Child has had mouth or dental surgery.
- Child has a congested nose.
- Child has breathing difficulty.
- Child is uncooperative (upset, drugged, extremely sleepy, or mentally retarded and unable to understand or follow instructions).
- Child is having a seizure.
- Doctor prefers another method.

Rectal Method

1. Use a rectal thermometer. (The type will be labeled on the package. Many rectal thermometers have a red color at the flat end. The silver-tipped end is short and round.) (Figure 5)
2. "Shake down" the thermometer so that the mercury (interior silver-colored line) is no higher than 94°F.
3. Apply petroleum jelly to the silver-colored tip of the thermometer.
4. Place the child on her abdomen and hold her firmly with one hand.
5. Insert the thermometer into the rectum about $\frac{1}{2}$ inch deep for an infant and about 1 inch deep for a child over 1 year. Hold the child firmly and hold the thermometer in place the entire time. (Figure 6)
6. Watch the mercury rise. If it does not move, gently push the thermometer in a little farther until the mercury does start to rise, and then hold the thermometer in place.
7. Remove the thermometer after 1 minute or after the mercury stops rising. (This may take 2 minutes.)

Axillary Method

1. Use an oral or rectal thermometer. (Figures 3, 5)
2. "Shake down" the thermometer so that the mercury (interior silver-colored line) is no higher than 94°F.
3. Raise the child's arm and place the silver-tipped end inside her armpit.
4. Lower the child's arm and hold it firmly against her body. (Figure 7)
5. Continue to hold the arm down; talk to or distract the child to keep her still.
6. Remove the thermometer after 5 minutes.

Measuring Method: Rectal

When to Use

- Child is 1 month or older.
- Child is unconscious.
- Child is uncooperative (will not keep mouth closed or may bite on thermometer if in mouth).
- Child is in shock.
- Child is experiencing hypothermia.
- Child had a seizure.
- Child feels very hot or has been running a fever. This method gives you the most accurate reading.
- Doctor prefers this method.

When Not to Use

- Child has diarrhea.
- Child has bad diaper rash with open sores on the skin.
- Child has burns or other injury or has had surgery near the rectum.
- Child has a history of a blood problem (for example, hemophilia, leukemia, anemia).

Figure 5

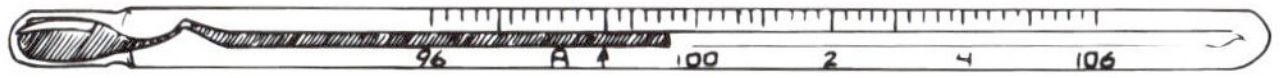

rectal thermometer

Figure 6

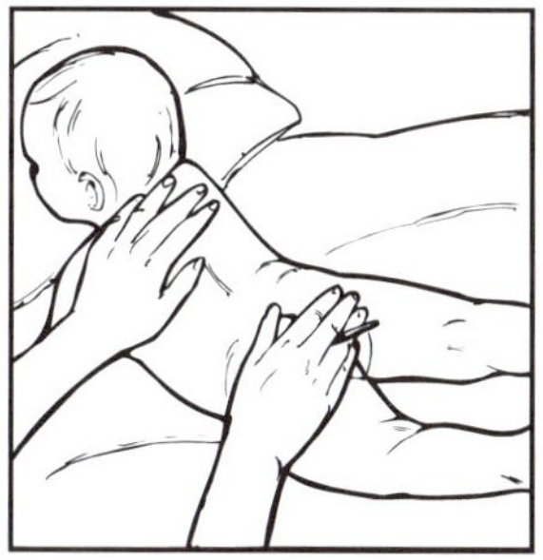

Figure 7

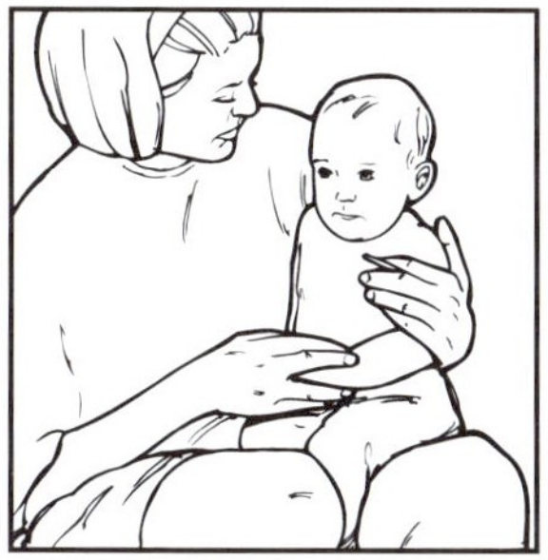

VITAL SIGNS

Measuring Method: Axillary

When to Use

- Child is any age, but this method is better for infants and not as dependable as other methods with older children.
- Other methods are not allowed by the child's doctor.

When Not to Use

- Child is in shock. All the blood is going to the heart, lungs, and brain to keep them healthy. The skin will be cold and will not give a true sign of blood temperature.
- Child is experiencing hypothermia, or subnormal temperature due to exposure to cold. The skin will be cold and will not give a true sign of blood temperature.
- Doctor prefers another method.

To Read the Thermometer

1. Wipe off the tip of the thermometer with a facial tissue (no water).
2. Turn the thermometer slowly until you can see the mercury (silver-colored line) inside. Look to see at which number the line ends. (Figure 8)
3. The longest line on the thermometer represents the first number in the temperature reading (for example, 96, 97, or 98 degrees). The short line represents tenths of a degree, the number after the decimal point in a temperature reading (for example, 98.6, 100.4, or 102.8 degrees). Each short line equals *two* tenths, so count the short lines as 100.2, 100.4, 100.6, 100.8, 101, 101.2, 101.4, 101.6, 101.8, 102 degrees, and so on.

Figure 8

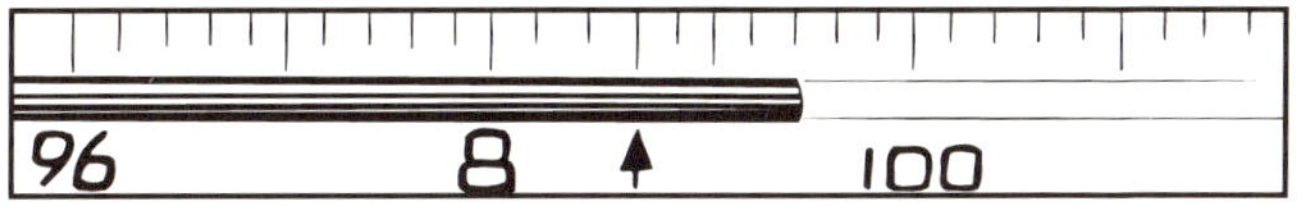

Ear thermometers work very quickly—usually in just a few seconds—are easy to read, and cause very little discomfort. Such a thermometer is accurate, but does require practice to insert and use correctly. Ear thermometers cost much more than glass or digital thermometers, with a usual starting price of $100.

When to Call the Doctor

Doctors differ in how and at what point they want a fever controlled. Ask the child's doctor about his or her recommendations. Some general guidelines with which most pediatricians agree are as follows.

Call the child's doctor if

- Child is under 4 months and either rectal or axillary temperature is over 100°F.
- Child is between 4 months and 2 years and either rectal or axillary temperature is over 102°F.
- Child has a fever between 105° and 106°F that cannot be brought down by acetaminophen.
- The child has a fever of 106°F or over.
- The child has any temperature 1–2 degrees above normal for 24 hours.
- The child has any fever and
  - —is extremely irritable or much more tired or sleepy than usual.
  - —has difficulty breathing.
  - —has a stiff neck. (She cries loudly if you try to bend her head forward, she holds her neck straight, or she complains of pain in her neck.)
  - —is having a seizure.
  - —pulls her ear or complains of ear pain.
  - —develops a rash.

— will not eat.
— has not passed any urine for 12 hours.
— complains of pain when she passes urine or suddenly has to pass urine much more frequently than usual.
— complains of a sore throat.

With any serious illness or injury, you must be sure to take care of the child's most life-threatening problems first. If you become involved in rescue breathing and/or cardiopulmonary resuscitation (CPR), you must continue to perform these procedures until the child's breathing and/or pulse return before proceeding to further steps. If available, an assistant may perform Steps 4 and 5 of the **Life-Threat Checklist** while you continue rescue breathing and/or CPR.

NOTE: *Suspect a back or neck injury if the child is unconscious and/or there was a major fall, a severe blow to the head, or a violent twisting or backward motion of the neck or back. Handle the child very carefully. Do not bend or twist her back or neck. Move the child only if her life is in danger, such as by fire or explosion, or if she is not breathing or has no pulse. See* ***Back and Neck Injuries,*** *page 47,* *for moving techniques.*

Step 1: Is the Child Conscious?

To check

a. Tap or gently shake the child's shoulder.

b. Call the child's name loudly. The child should respond either verbally or physically if conscious.

Yes

Proceed to Step 2.

No

a. If a back or neck injury is suspected, handle the child carefully without bending or twisting the back or neck.

b. Shout for help. Have the helper **call 911 or the rescue squad.**

c. If the child is:

0–8 years, and no help is available, stay with the child and proceed to Step 2.

8+ years, **call 911 or the rescue squad.** Proceed to Step 2.

Step 3: Is the Child's Heart Beating?

To check

a. Use your index and middle fingers.

b. For an infant, 0–1 year, check inside the upper arm, between the elbow and armpit. For a child older than 1 year, check the side of the neck, below the angle of the jaw.

c. Check for 5–10 seconds. Move your fingers slightly to find the correct location if you do not feel a pulse within 3 seconds. See **Checking Pulse,** page 13, for more details, if necessary.

Yes

a. Have someone **call 911 or the rescue squad** if you have not already done so. If you are alone, call after you perform rescue breathing for 1 minute.

b. Continue rescue breathing until the child breathes on her own or medical assistance arrives.

c. Another person may proceed with Steps 4 and 5.

No

a. Have someone **call 911 or the rescue squad** if you have not already done so. If you are alone, call after you perform cardiopulmonary resuscitation (CPR) for 1 minute.

b. Begin CPR. See **Rescue Breathing/ Cardiopulmonary Resuscitation (CPR):** 0–1 year, page 27; 1–8 years, page 33; 8+ years, page 39.

c. Another person may proceed with Steps 4 and 5.

Step 4: Is There Obvious Bleeding?

Yes

a. Control the bleeding. See **Bleeding and Cuts,** page 63. If a bone may be broken, see **Bleeding and Cuts: If a Fracture is Suspected,** page 65. If there is a puncture or stab wound, see **Puncture Wounds,** page 159.

b. Proceed to Step 5.

No

Proceed to Step 5.

Step 5: Is the Child in Shock?

Signs of shock:

- Cold, moist skin.
- Rapid, faint pulse.
- Pale or "purplish" skin.
- Pale or blue lips, gums, or nails.
- Weakness; fainting.
- Weak, rapid, and shallow breathing; or deep but irregular breathing; or gasping.
- Restlessness; anxiety.
- Extreme thirst.
- Nausea.

Yes

a. Treat for shock. See **Shock,** page 169.

b. **Call 911 or the rescue squad** if you have not already done so.

c. Monitor breathing and pulse. If necessary, see **Rescue Breathing/Cardiopulmonary Resuscitation (CPR):** 0–1 year, page 27; 1–8 years, page 33; 8+ years, page 39.

No

a. Treat for shock if the child has suffered any type of serious illness or injury (trauma, burn, poisoning, drug overdose, and so on); was without oxygen for any length of time (suffocation, drowning, smoke or poisonous gas inhalation); has had a severe allergic reaction to a food, medication, or insect bite; or has had a severe emotional reaction to a stressful event. Treat even before symptoms appear, to help prevent shock. See **Shock,** page 169.

b. If any events listed above have occurred, **call 911 or the rescue squad** if you have not already done so.

c. If the child is unconscious but breathing, place the child in the recovery position, as described in **Rescue Breathing/Cardiopulmonary Resuscitation (CPR),** Step 5: 0–1 year, page 27; 1–8 years, page 33; 8+ years, page 39.

Step 6: Proceed to Part III

After you have attended to the child's most life-threatening problems, proceed to the instructions specific to the type of injury or illness the child has sustained.

1. Check the infant's response to stimulation.

a. Tap or gently shake the infant's shoulder; call his name loudly and take note of any signs of response. (Figure 1)

b. If there is a possibility of a back or neck injury, pinch his skin instead.

2. Call out for help.

Have someone come to your side in case you need help, but do not leave the infant to get help.

3. Position the infant on his back.

a. Place the infant on his back on a firm, flat surface. (Figure 2)

b. If there is a possibility of a back or neck injury, see **Back and Neck Injuries,** page 45, for positioning.

c. Open the child's clothing to reveal his chest.

4. Open the airway.

a. If you do not suspect a back or neck injury, lift the infant's chin up gently with one hand while pushing down on his forehead with your other hand. His head should be in a neutral position, and the neck should not be stretched far back. The corner of his mouth should be in a straight line with the middle of his ear. (Figure 3)

Figure 1

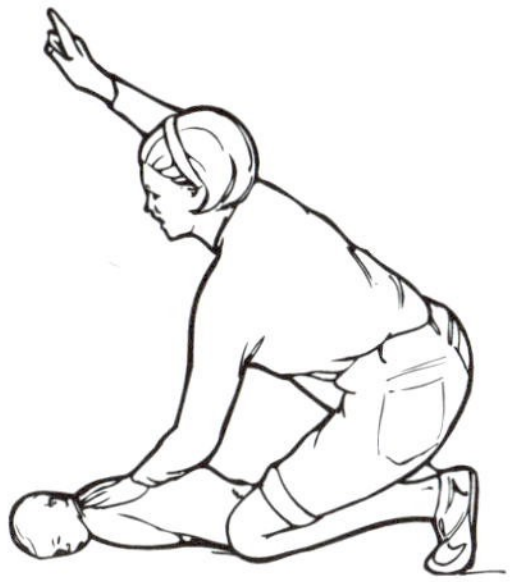

Figure 2

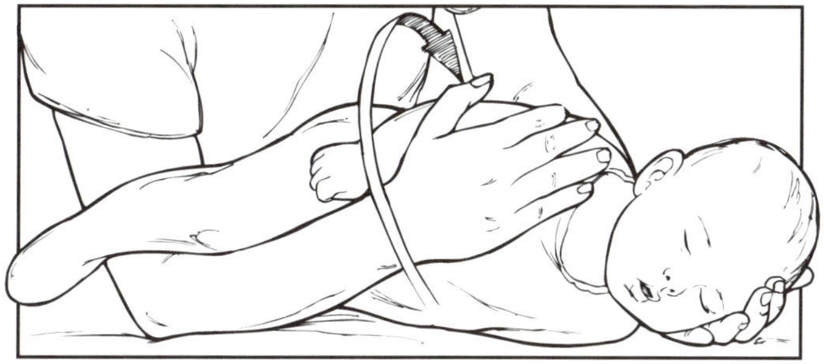

Figure 3

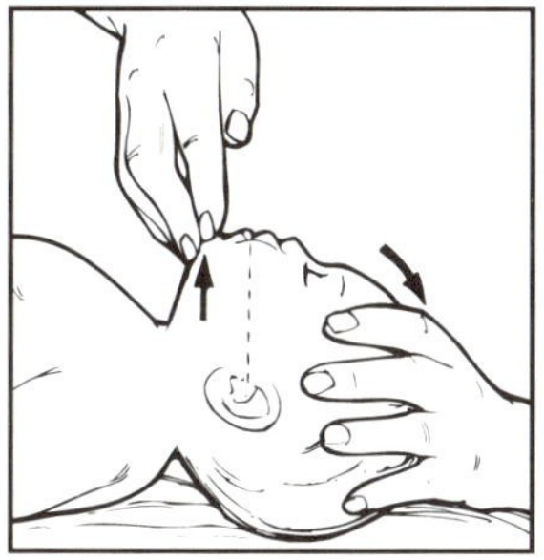

Each breath should be 1 to 1½ seconds long, with a pause between breaths in which you allow the chest to fall and air to leave the lungs. (Figure 7)

If the infant's chest does not rise, and/or your breath does not go in easily,

a. Reposition the infant's head, lift his chin, and try again. His tongue may have been blocking the airway.

b. If you still cannot get air in, the airway may be blocked by an object. Follow the instructions in **Choking,** page 97. Start with Step 8.

6. Check the infant's pulse.

a. Keep one hand on the infant's forehead to keep the airway open.

b. Find the infant's pulse using your index and middle fingers on the inside of his upper arm, between the elbow and armpit. Press gently. Allow 5–10 seconds to feel the pulse. You may have to move your fingers slightly to find the pulse. Do not rush—a very weak pulse may be hard to feel. Concentrate. (Figure 8)

c. Once you have determined the infant's pulse, have someone **call 911 or the rescue squad.** If you are alone, stay with the infant.

If a pulse is present but the infant is still not breathing, continue rescue breathing. Give one breath every 3 seconds.

a. Count "1-and-2-and-3-and," breathe, count "1-and-2-and-3-and," breathe, and so on. (Figure 7, above)

b. Perform rescue breathing for 1 minute, then recheck breathing.

Figure 7

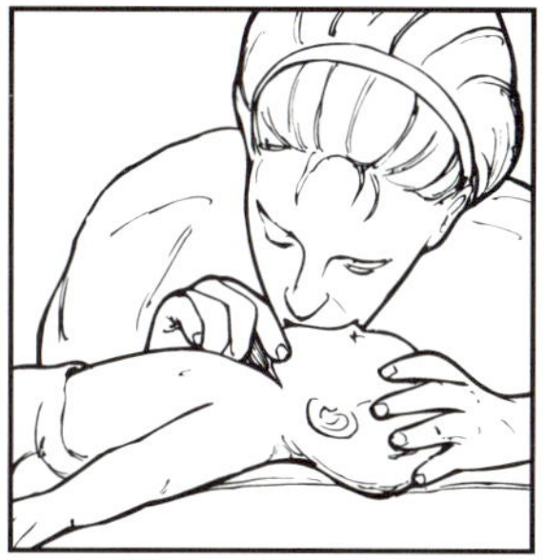

Figure 8

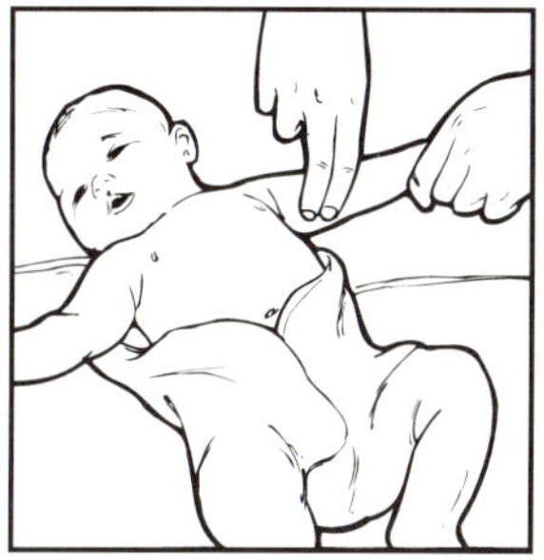

c. If you are alone, **call 911 or the rescue squad** now.

d. Return to the infant, and recheck breathing and pulse.

e. Continue rescue breathing until medical help arrives or the infant begins breathing on his own. Recheck breathing every few minutes during rescue breathing.

If there is no pulse, find the location for chest compressions.

a. Remove the infant's shirt.

b. Keep one hand on the infant's forehead to keep his head still and to keep the airway open throughout CPR.

c. Place the index finger of your other hand in the center of his chest, on his breastbone between his nipples; point the index finger toward his arm.

d. Place your next two fingers next to your index finger. All three fingers should point toward the infant's arm. (Figure 9)

e. Raise your index finger off his chest. (Figure 10) If you have a large hand, or the infant is very small, your fingers may be at the bottom tip of the breast-bone, which can be felt. Move them up toward his head slightly, off the breastbone tip so you do not break it.

f. Once in the correct position on the breastbone, do not move your two fingers from it.

7. Begin chest compressions.

a. With your two fingers, press downward, toward the infant's back, $\frac{1}{2}$ to 1 inch. Use short, smooth, quick strokes. Press down five times, allowing his chest to come up completely each time before pressing down again. Count "1-2-3-4-5" as you press (five compressions in 3 seconds). (Figure 11)

Figure 9

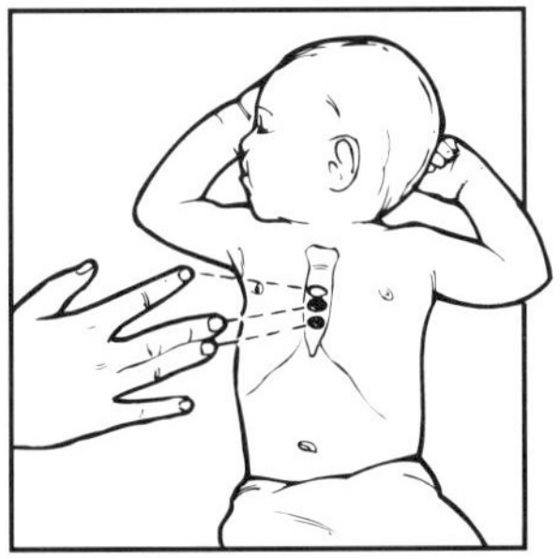

Figure 10

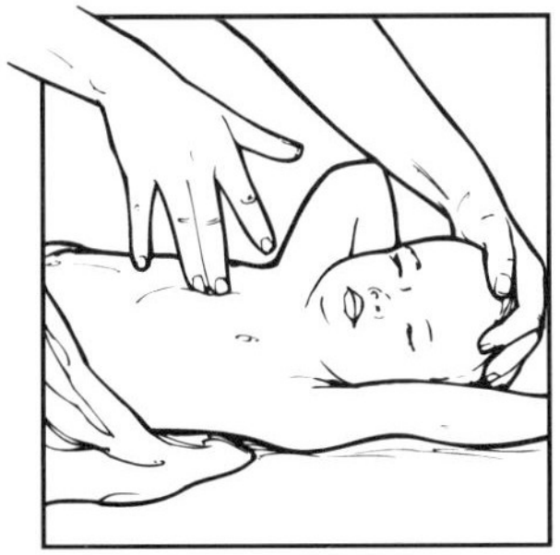

Figure 11

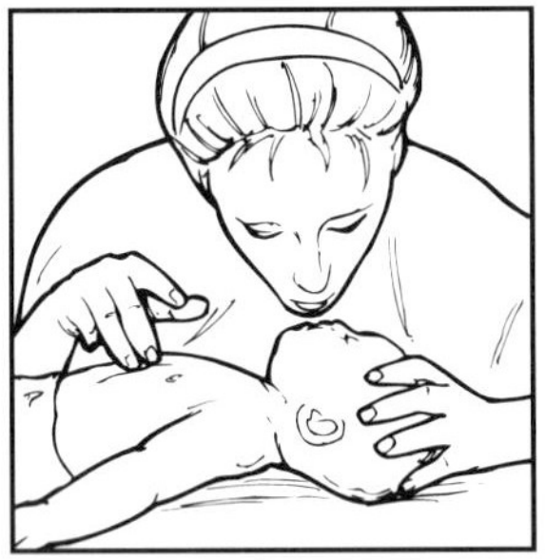

b. As your fingers are coming up after "5," give one breath. Do not pause or slow down. Do not take your fingers off his chest.

c. Continue the cycle of five compressions and one breath. Press down while counting "1-2-3-4-5," then one breath, then press down while counting "1-2-3-4-5," then one breath, and so on. You should be performing at a rate of one hundred compressions and twenty breaths per minute. (Infants have faster heart and breathing rates than adults.)

8. After twenty cycles, or approximately 1 minute, recheck pulse and breathing for 5 seconds.

(Figure 12)

Figure 12

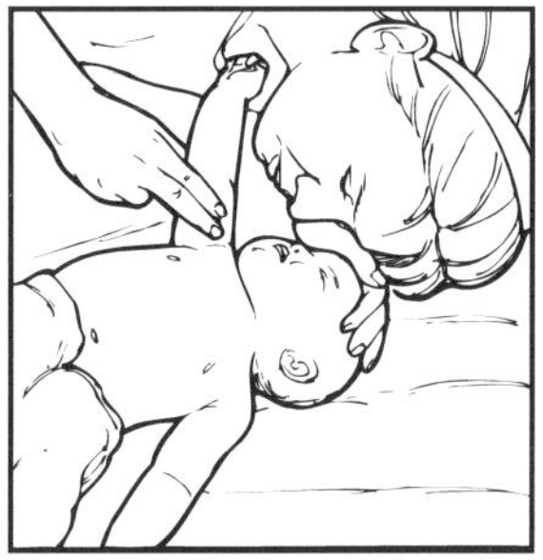

9. If you are alone, call 911 or the rescue squad now.

10. Return to the infant and recheck breathing and pulse.

Carefully monitor the child.

If there is a pulse but no breathing, continue rescue breathing at the rate of one breath every 3 seconds until medical help arrives or breathing returns.

(Figure 13)

Recheck the infant's breathing every few minutes. Stop rescue breathing if he breathes on his own, but continue to observe.

Figure 13

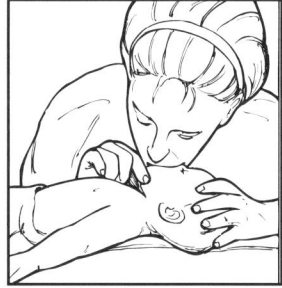

Small Children 1–8 Years

1. Check the child's response to stimulation.

a. Tap or gently shake the child's shoulder; call her name loudly and take note of any signs of response. (Figure 1)

b. If there is a possibility of a back or neck injury, pinch her skin instead.

2. Call out for help.

Have someone come to your side in case you need help, but do not leave the child to get help.

3. Position the child on her back.

a. Place the child on her back on a firm, flat surface. (Figure 2)

b. If there is a possibility of a back or neck injury, see **Back and Neck Injuries,** page 45, for positioning.

c. Open the child's clothing to reveal her chest.

4. Open the airway.

a. If you do not suspect a back or neck injury, lift the child's chin up gently with one hand while pushing down on her forehead with your other hand. Lift her chin so the teeth are brought almost together, but do not close the mouth. Her head should be in a neutral position, and the neck should not be stretched far back. (Figure 3)

Figure 1

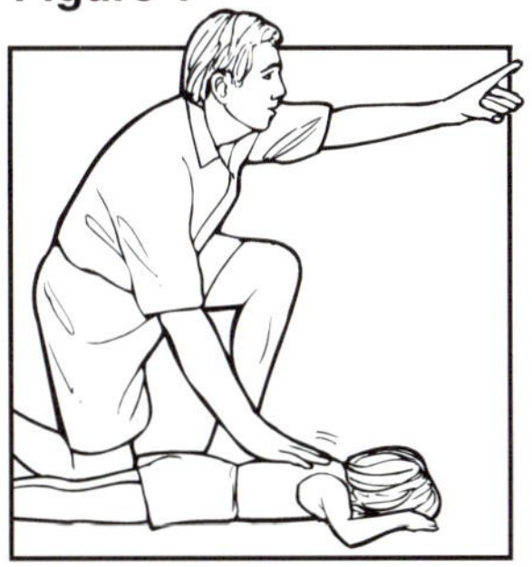

Figure 2

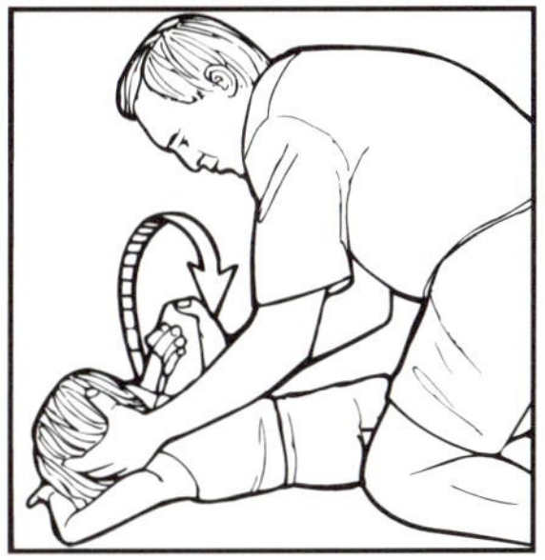

Figure 3

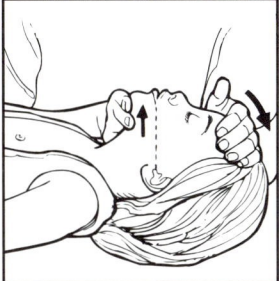

b. If there is a possibility of a back or neck injury, do not bend her neck or tilt her head back. Place two or three fingers under each side of her lower jaw and lift upward (jaw-thrust technique). (Figure 4)

5. Check the child's breathing.

Look at her chest; listen and feel for air from her mouth or nose. Check for 3–5 seconds. (Figure 5)

If the child is breathing but not responsive,

a. Position her head to keep the airway open. Use the jaw-thrust technique if there is a possibility of a back or neck injury.

b. If a back or neck injury is not suspected, place the child in the recovery position, as follows:

1. Kneel beside the child.
2. Turn the child onto her side by pulling her toward you.
3. Position the child's head to keep the airway open.
4. Support her body by bending the arm and leg nearest to you. (Figure 6)

c. Call 911 or the rescue squad.

d. Return to the child and await medical assistance. Continue to observe her breathing. If breathing stops, follow instructions below.

If the child is not breathing, give two rescue breaths.

a. Keep one hand on her forehead to keep the airway open. With the index finger and thumb of that hand, pinch the child's nose closed.

b. Take in a deep breath.

Figure 4

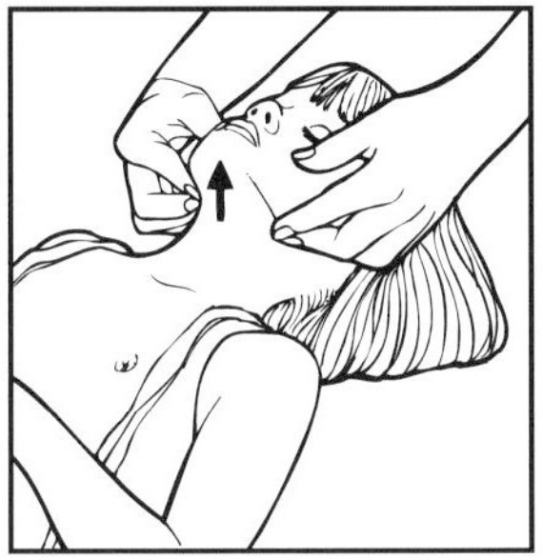

Figure 5

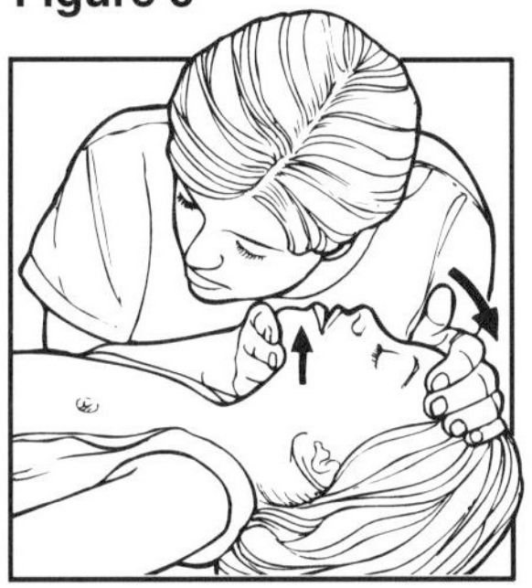

Figure 6

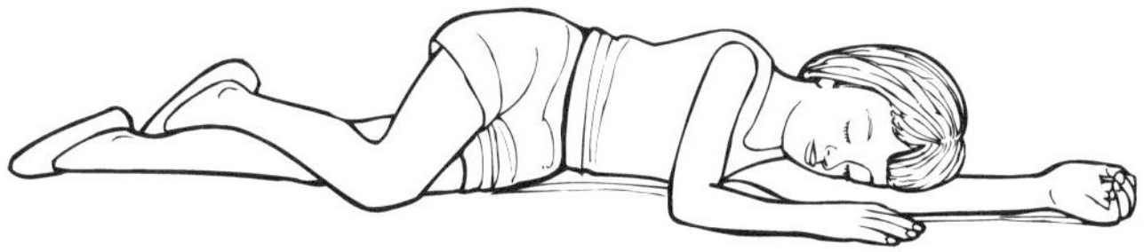

c. Completely and tightly cover the child's mouth with your mouth. (Figure 7)

d. Give two breaths, using only enough force to make the child's chest rise. (Look at her chest from the corner of your eye.) Each breath should be 1 to $1\frac{1}{2}$ seconds long, with a pause between breaths in which you allow the chest to fall and air to leave the lungs.

Figure 7

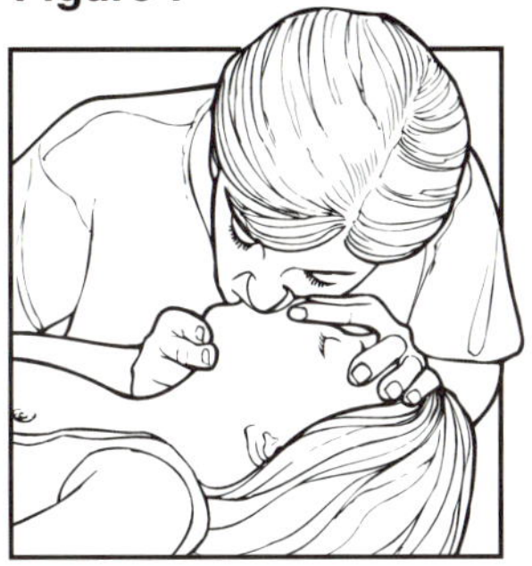

If the child's chest does not rise, and/or your breath does not go in easily,

a. Reposition the child's head, lift her chin, and try again. Her tongue may have been blocking the airway.

b. If you still cannot get air in, the airway may be blocked by an object. Follow the instructions in **Choking,** page 109. Start with Step 8.

6. Check the child's pulse.

a. Keep one hand on the child's forehead to keep the airway open.

b. Place the index and middle fingers of your other hand in the middle of her neck, on the Adam's apple (the firm, bulging area).

c. Slide the two fingers toward you into the groove on the side of the neck, below the angle or "pointy" part of the jaw. (Figure 8)

d. Press gently with your fingertips. Allow 5–10 seconds to feel the pulse. You may have to move your fingers slightly to find the pulse. Do not rush—a very weak pulse may be hard to feel. Concentrate.

e. Have someone **call 911 or the rescue squad.** If you are alone, stay with the child.

Figure 8

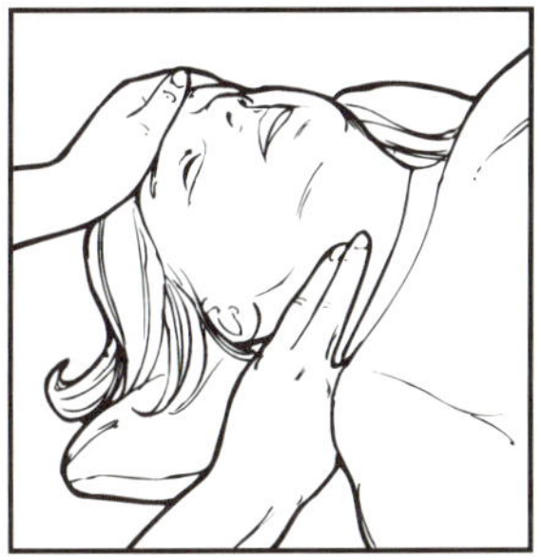

7. Begin chest compressions.

a. Keeping your fingers off the child's chest, press with the heel of your hand directly downward, toward the child's back. Press down 1 to 1½ inches. Use smooth, even strokes. Your shoulders should be over the child's breastbone, with your arm straight. Press down five times, allowing her chest to come up completely before pressing down again. Count "1-2-3-4-5" as you press (five compressions in 3 seconds). (Figure 11)

b. After the fifth compression, give one breath. Leave your hand on the child's chest. If your hand comes off the child's chest, find the correct location again before replacing it.

c. Continue the cycle of five compressions and one breath. Press down while counting "1-2-3-4-5," then breathe, then press down while counting "1-2-3-4-5," then breathe, and so on. You should be performing at a rate of one hundred compressions and twenty breaths per minute.

Figure 11

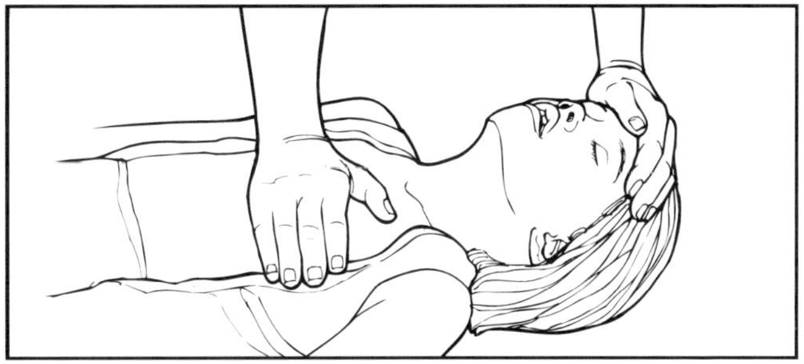

8. After twenty cycles, or approximately 1 minute, recheck pulse and breathing for 5 seconds.

(Figure 12)

Figure 12

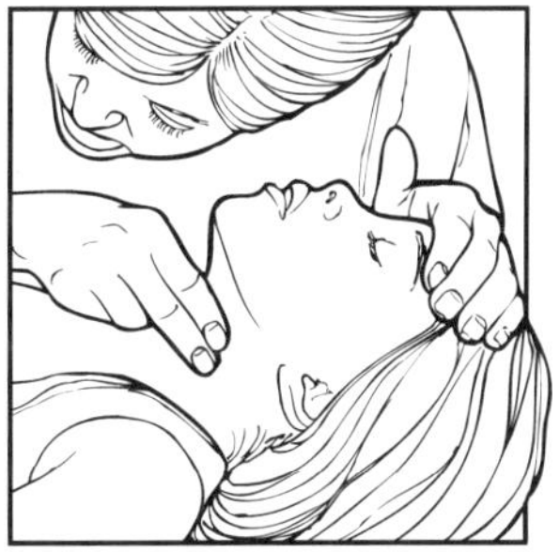

9. If you are alone, call 911 or the rescue squad now.

10. Return to the child and recheck breathing and pulse.

Carefully monitor the child.

If there is a pulse but no breathing, continue rescue breathing at the rate of one breath every 3 seconds until medical help arrives or breathing returns.

(Figure 13)

Recheck the child's breathing every few minutes. Stop rescue breathing if she breathes on her own, but continue to observe.

If there is no pulse and no breathing, continue CPR until medical help arrives or breathing and pulse return.

(Figure 14)

Recheck the child's breathing and pulse every few minutes. Continue CPR, or rescue breathing, as necessary.

Figure 13

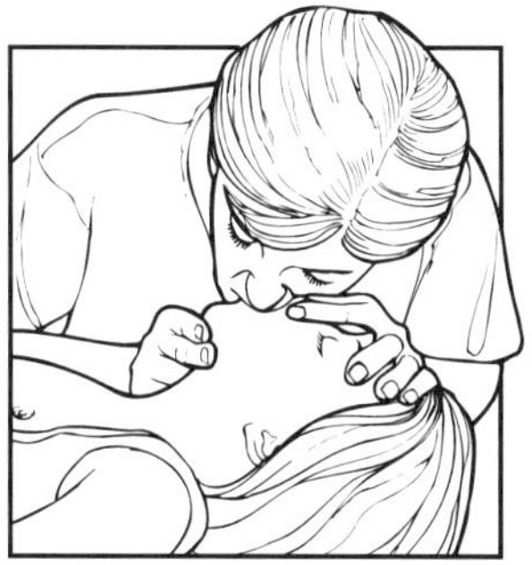

Figure 14

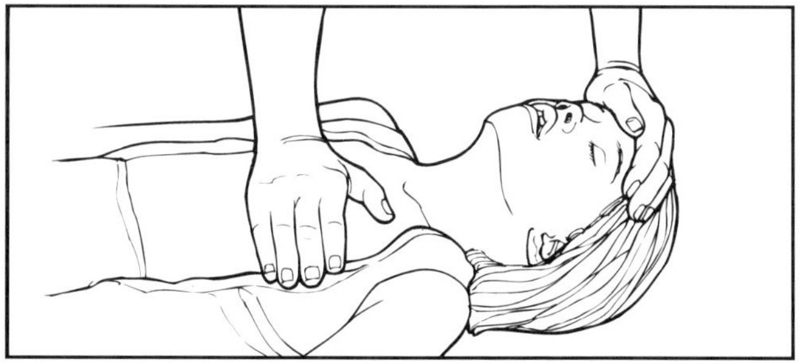

1. Check the child's response to stimulation.

a. Tap or gently shake the child's shoulder; call his name loudly and take note of any signs of response. (Figure 1)

b. If there is a possibility of a back or neck injury, pinch his skin instead.

2. Call 911 or the rescue squad.

The caller should

a. Give the address and phone number of your location. (Figure 2)

b. Describe what happened.

c. Listen for instructions.

d. Hang up only when told to do so by the operator.

NOTE: *In adult CPR (for persons older than 8 years) it is important to call 911 or the rescue squad as soon as you have determined that the victim is unconscious. Older children and adults often require the skills and equipment available only from emergency medical personnel. Infants and other young children, on the other hand, are often more in need of oxygen, which can be delivered immediately through rescue breathing or CPR performed by you. Medical assistance can then be sought after the first minute of rescue breathing or CPR.*

Figure 1

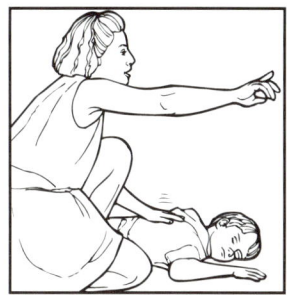

Figure 2

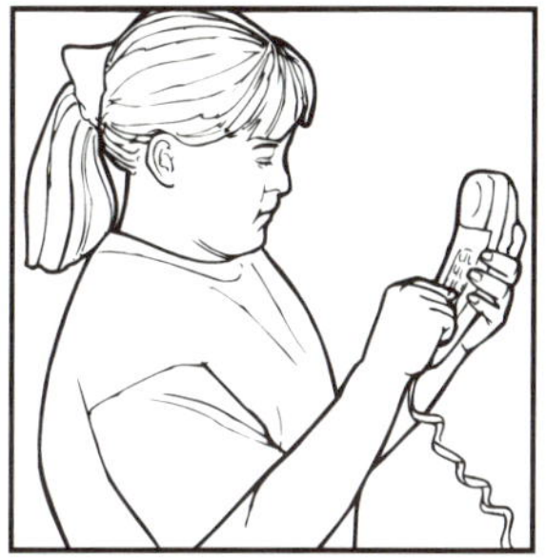

c. Stay with the child and await medical assistance. Continue to observe his breathing. If breathing stops, follow instructions below.

If the child is not breathing, give two rescue breaths.

a. Keep one hand on his forehead to keep the airway open. With the index finger and thumb of that hand, pinch the child's nose closed.

b. Take in a deep breath.

c. Completely and tightly cover the child's mouth with your mouth. (Figure 8)

d. Give two breaths, using only enough force to make the child's chest rise. (Look at his chest from the corner of your eye.) Each breath should be 1 to $1\frac{1}{2}$ seconds long, with a pause between breaths in which you allow the chest to fall and air to leave the lungs.

Figure 8

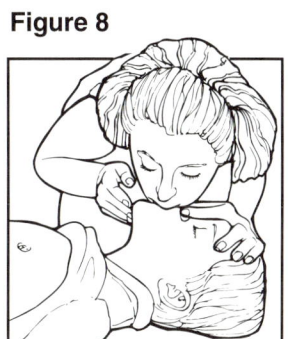

If the child's chest does not rise, and/or your breath does not go in easily,

a. Reposition the child's head, lift his chin, and try again. His tongue may have been blocking the airway.

b. If you still cannot get air in, the airway may be blocked by an object. Follow the instructions in **Choking,** page 109. Start with Step 8.

6. Check the child's pulse.

a. Keep one hand on the child's forehead to keep the airway open.

b. Place the index and middle fingers of your other hand in the middle of his neck, on the Adam's apple (the firm, bulging area).

c. Slide the two fingers toward you into the groove on the side of the neck, below the angle or "pointy" part of the jaw. (Figure 9)

d. Press gently with your fingertips. Allow 5–10 seconds to feel the pulse. You may have to move your fingers slightly to find the pulse. Do not rush—a very weak pulse may be hard to feel. Concentrate.

If a pulse is present but the child is still not breathing, continue rescue breathing. Give one breath every 5 seconds.

a. Count "1-and-2-and-3-and-4-and-5-and," breathe, count "1-and-2-and-3-and-4-and-5-and," breathe, and so on. (Figure 10)

b. Perform rescue breathing for 1 minute, then recheck breathing.

c. Continue rescue breathing until medical help arrives or the child begins breathing on his own. Recheck breathing every few minutes during rescue breathing.

If there is no pulse, find the location for chest compressions.

With the first two fingers of your left hand (your right hand if you are left-handed), find the bottom of the child's rib cage. Slide your fingers upward along the rib cage until you feel the tip of the breastbone in the center of the chest. Place the heel of your right hand next to your two fingers, higher on the breast bone. (Figure 11) Remove your two fingers from the child's chest. The heel of your hand should not be on the breastbone tip because you might break it. The fingers of your right hand should point toward the child's arm and should be up, off the chest.

Figure 9

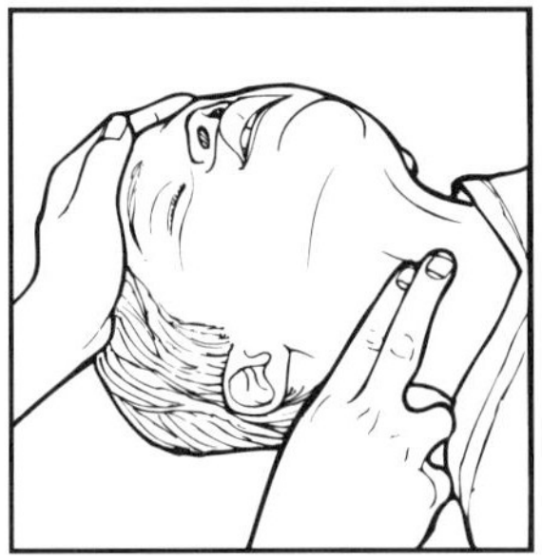

Figure 10

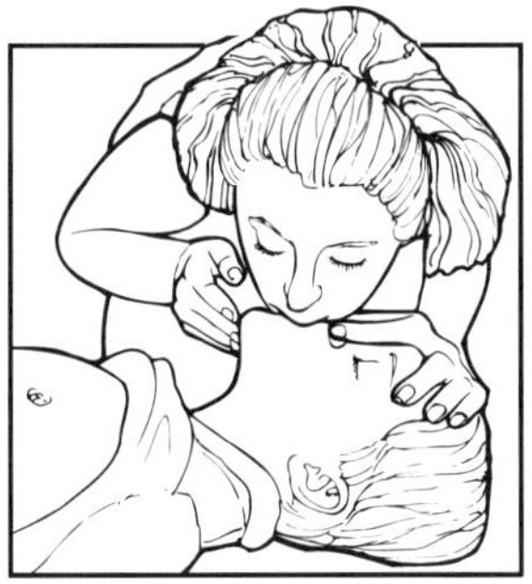

Figure 11

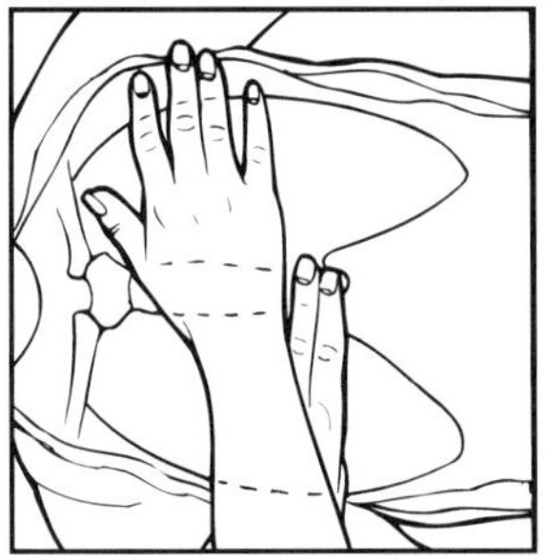

7. Begin chest compressions.

a. Place your other hand (left hand) on top of the hand you have on the child's chest (right hand).

b. Interlock the fingers of both hands so that your top fingers are holding your bottom fingers up, off the child's chest. (Figure 12) You should be up on your knees, with your shoulders directly over the child's breastbone. Your arms should be straight, with the elbows locked.

c. Press directly downward, toward the child's back, using your weight. Do not bend your arms. Adjust the force for the size of the child. Press down $1\frac{1}{2}$ to 2 inches. Use smooth, even strokes. Press down fifteen times, allowing the child's chest to come up completely before pressing down again. Count "1-2-3-4-5-...-15" as you press (fifteen compressions in 10 seconds). (Figure 13)

d. After the fifteenth compression, open the airway and give two breaths, $1\frac{1}{2}$ to 2 seconds each, pausing between each breath.

e. Continue the cycle of fifteen compressions and two breaths. Press down while counting "1-2-3-4-5-...-15," then breathe and pause, then breathe again, then press down while counting "1-2-3-4-5-...-15," then breathe and pause, then breathe again, and so on. You should be performing at a rate of eighty to one hundred compressions and twelve breaths per minute.

Figure 12

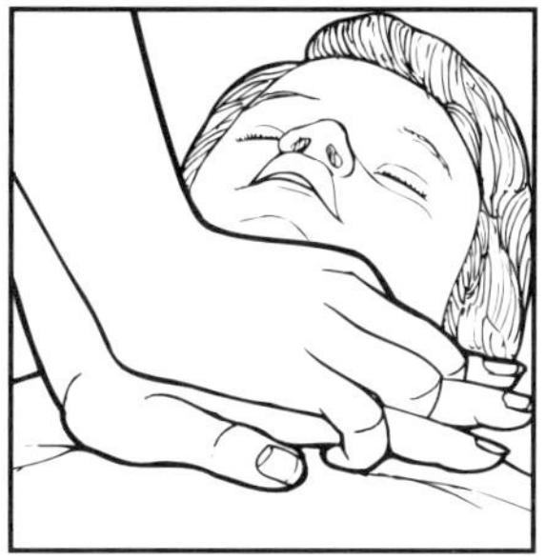

Figure 13

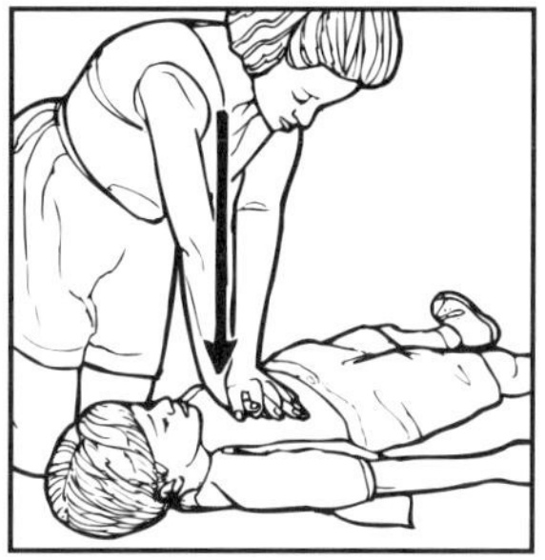

8. After four cycles, or approximately 1 minute, recheck pulse and breathing for 5 seconds.

(Figure 14)

Carefully monitor the child.

Figure 14

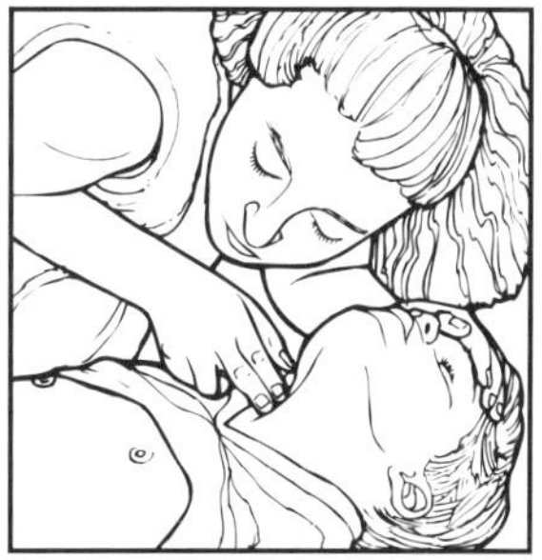

Safety Highlights

Do

- **Do** assume the child has a back or neck injury if there has been a severe blow to the head.
- **Do** assume the child has a back or neck injury if the child is unconscious and the surroundings indicate trauma to the back, neck, or head.

Don't

- **Don't** assume the child is okay just because he or she has some movement or feeling; a spinal cord injury can take minutes to hours to develop.
- **Don't** move the child unless absolutely necessary. See **Moving a Child in an Emergency Situation,** page 47.

Immediate Action

1. Look at the surroundings and the general appearance of the child.

(Take a few seconds.)

Do not move the child.

- Was the child's head hit forcibly by a blunt object? (Either the head was struck by an object or the head struck an object with force when the child dove into a pool, hit a wall, or was thrown from a vehicle or bicycle.) (Figure 1)
- Was the child's head thrown back violently?
- If the child is an infant, was he violently shaken?
- Is the child lying with his body in a twisted position?

If the answer to any of these questions is *yes,* the child may have a back or neck injury. Handle him carefully. Do not bend or twist his neck or body.

Figure 1

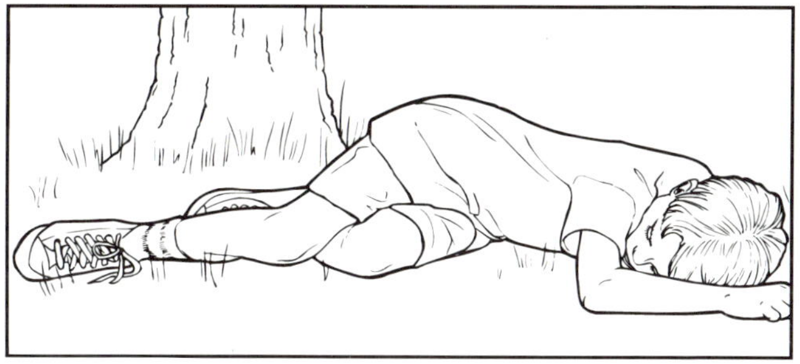

2. Check for and treat the most life-threatening problems now.

Check for signs of unconsciousness, no breathing, no pulse, bleeding, and shock. (Figure 2) See **Life-Threat Checklist,** page 23. **Call 911 or the rescue squad** as recommended in **Life-Threat Checklist.**

Once the most life-threatening problems have been attended to, you may proceed with further treatment as instructed below.

Figure 2

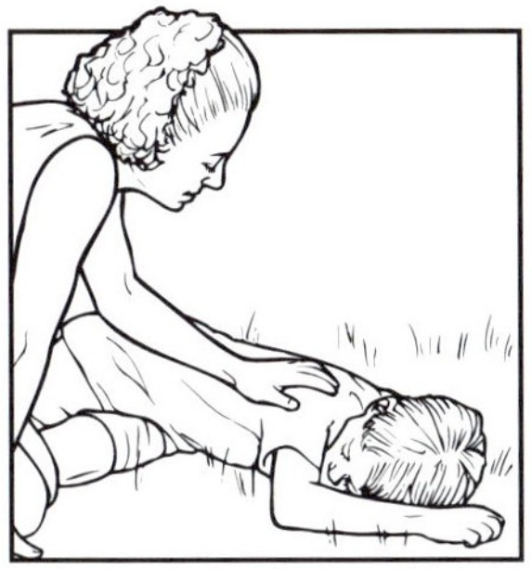

BACK AND NECK INJURIES

3. Check the child for signs of a back or neck injury:

- Twisted body
- Cuts or bruises on the head, face, shoulders, back, or abdomen
- Unconsciousness—does not respond when his shoulder is gently shaken or when his name is called loudly
- Difficult or no breathing
- Inability to move one or more body parts (may occur slowly, over hours)
- Pain in the back or neck
- Numbness or tingling in an arm or leg (if child is conscious; may occur slowly, over hours)
- Inability to feel it when you gently touch his hands, arms, legs, or feet
- Loss of bowel or bladder control (not a reliable sign in a young child who is not yet toilet trained)

4. If a back or neck injury is suspected, call 911 or the rescue squad if you have not already done so.

5. Prevent the child from moving.

Immobilize the child in the position you found him. Place rolled blankets, clothing, or newspapers around the child's head and along the sides of his neck and body. Keep them in place with heavy objects, such as stones, bricks, or books. (Figure 3, 4)

6. Monitor the child's breathing and pulse.

a. Keep the airway open using the jaw-thrust technique. Do not bend the neck or tilt the head back. Place two or three fingers under each side of the lower jaw and lift upward. (Figure 5)

b. If breathing stops, begin rescue breathing. See **Rescue Breathing/Cardiopulmonary Resuscitation (CPR):** 0–1 year, page 27; 1–8 years, page 33; 8+ years, page 39.

c. If the child's heart stops, begin CPR. See **Rescue Breathing/Cardiopulmonary Resuscitation (CPR):** 0–1 year, page 27; 1–8 years, page 33; 8+ years, page 39.

Figure 3

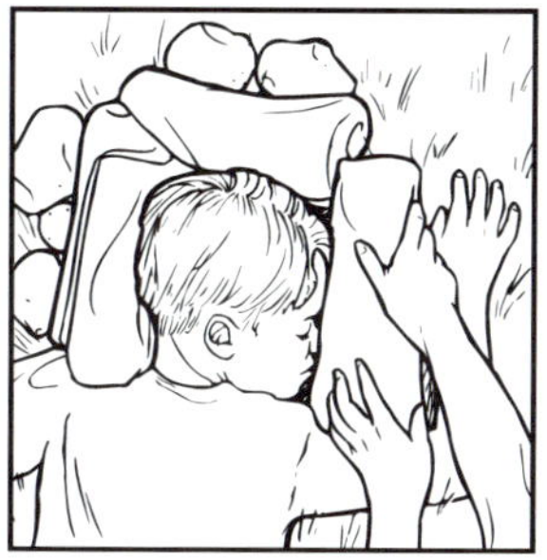

Figure 4

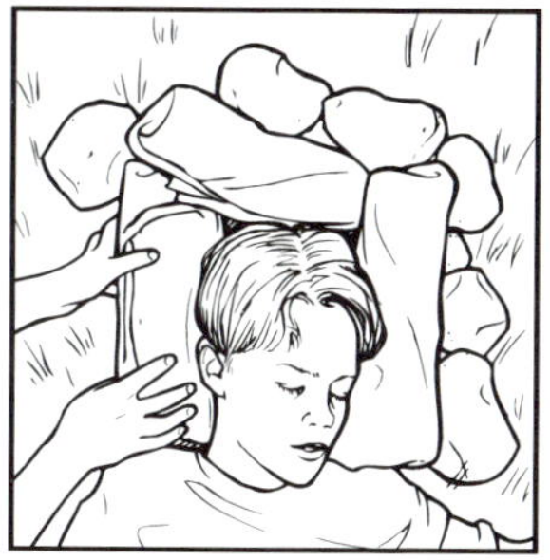

Figure 5

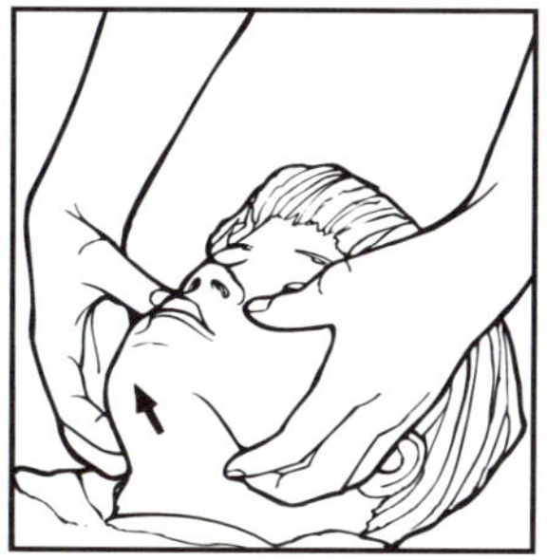

Moving a Child in an Emergency Situation

If a back or neck injury is suspected, you may have to move the child because:

- His life is threatened by fire, explosion, or other danger before medical help can arrive.
- He is lying face down and is not breathing and/or has no pulse.
- He is vomiting or is bleeding from the mouth.

If the Child Is on His Back and You Have Help

Follow these instructions if a blanket, coat, board, or ironing board is available; if not available, follow the instructions above. Use at least three people—one to support the child's head in the position found, one at his shoulders, and at least one to support his waist and legs. The person positioned at the head should count and give the command to roll the child onto his side. Roll him as a unit while keeping him straight. (Figure 10) Slide a blanket, coat, board, or ironing board next to the child and then roll him as a unit onto his back on top of the blanket, coat, board, or ironing board. (Figure 8, above) Carry the child to safety. Keep his head and neck well supported at all times.

Figure 10

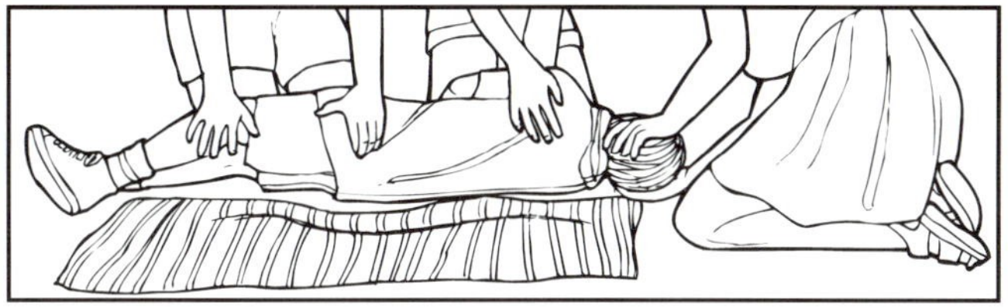

If the Child Is in a Car Seat

a. Leave the child strapped into the car seat.

b. Remove the car seat from the car. (Figure 11)

c. Await medical assistance, observing the child for signs of breathing difficulty, bleeding, or a change in level of consciousness. If the child must be removed from the car seat to administer rescue breathing or CPR, remove her gently, keeping her head and neck in line with the rest of her body.

Figure 11

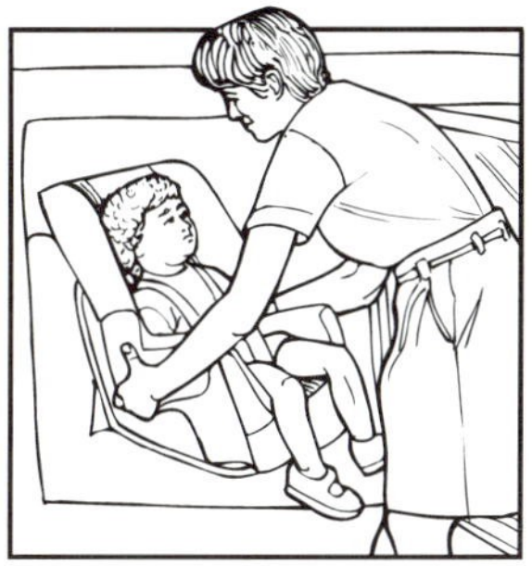

If the Child Is Lying Face Down and Is Not Breathing or Has No Pulse

If You Are Alone

Roll the child onto his back, as follows. Reach across the child and place your hand under the arm farthest away from you. Support the child's head with your other hand. Slowly pull the child toward you without allowing his head to move. Continue to slowly turn the child onto his back. (Figure 12) See **Rescue Breathing/Cardiopulmonary Resuscitation (CPR),** immediately: 0–1 year, page 27; 1–8 years, page 33; 8+ years, page 39.

Figure 12

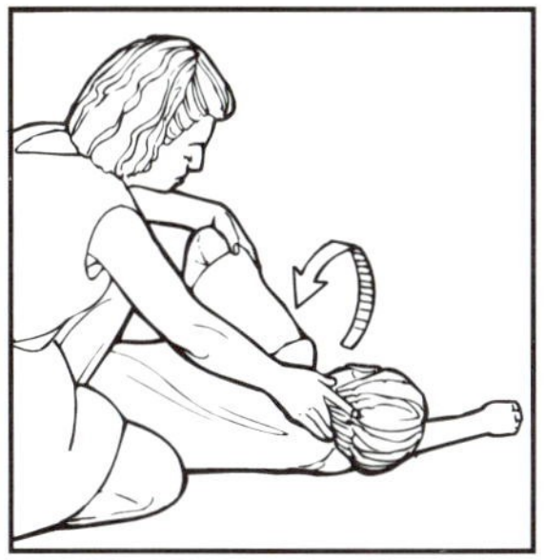

If You Have Help

Use at least three people—one to support the child's head in the position found, one at his shoulders, and at least one to support his waist and legs. The person positioned at the head should count and give the command to roll the child onto his side. (Figure 13) Roll him as a unit while keeping him straight. Keep his head and neck well supported at all times. See **Rescue Breathing/Cardiopulmonary Resuscitation (CPR),** immediately: 0–1 year, page 27; 1–8 years, page 33; 8+ years, page 39.

Figure 13

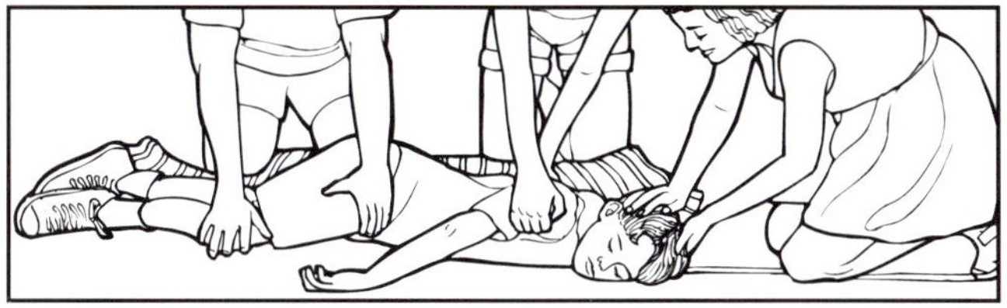

If the Child Is Vomiting or Is Bleeding From the Mouth

If You Are Alone

Seek help to turn the child onto his side for maximum safety. If no help is available, first secure a blanket. Then, reach across the child and place your hand under the arm farthest away from you. Support the child's head with your other hand. Slowly and cautiously pull the child toward you, turning him onto his side, without allowing his head to move. Support his head at all times and turn him as a unit. Stay with the child, supporting his head by holding it in place until medical help arrives. Do not allow the head or neck to move; if available, place blankets, pillows, or clothing beneath his head and neck to provide extra support. (Figure 14) Clear the mouth of blood or vomit. Cover the child with the blanket. Keep the airway open by holding the head in a straight position.

Figure 14

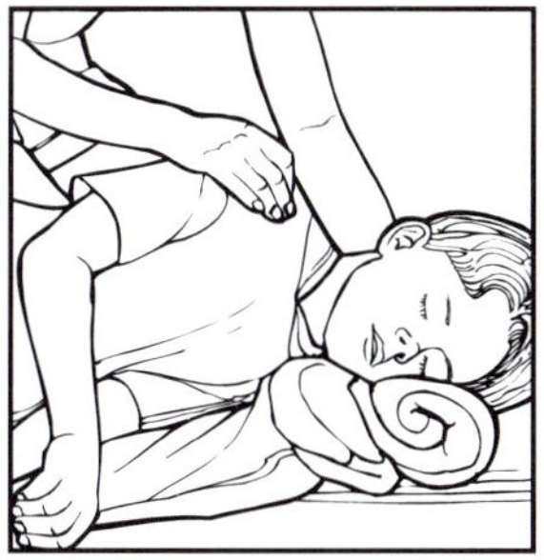

If You Have Help

To turn the child onto his side, use at least three people—one to support the child's head in the position found, one at his shoulders, and at least one to support his waist and legs. The person positioned at the head should count and give the command to roll the child onto his side. (Figure 13) Roll him as a unit while keeping him straight. Keep his head and neck well supported at all times. Stay with the child, supporting his head by holding it in place until medical help arrives. Do not allow the head or neck to move; if available, place blankets, pillows, or clothing beneath his head and neck to provide extra support. (Figure 14, above) One person can support the head, and other available people can support the back and legs. Clear the mouth of blood or vomit. Cover the child with a blanket. Keep the airway open by holding the head in a straight position.

When to See a Doctor

If a back or neck injury is suspected, the child should be transported to a medical facility by ambulance.

Home Treatment

A back or neck injury can be life threatening and must not be treated at home.

Safety Highlights

Do

- **Do** suspect rabies in wild animals, especially skunks, foxes, bats, raccoons, and opossums. (Rabbits and rodents do not get rabies.)
- **Do** report signs of wound infection or of illness to the doctor.
- **Do** act in a calm manner to prevent anxiety in the child.

Don't

- **Don't** apply direct pressure on a wound if a fracture (broken bone) is suspected.
- **Don't** apply a bandage so tightly that the area past the bandage turns blue, cold, or numb.
- **Don't** use iodine, merbromin (for example, Mercurochrome®), or other antiseptics without first checking with the doctor.

Immediate Action

1. Control any bleeding.

See **Bleeding and Cuts,** page 63.

2. Check the wound for signs of a bite:

- Broken skin, tears, or deep puncture marks
- Heavy or uncontrollable bleeding (see **Bleeding and Cuts,** page 63)
- Signs of a fracture (broken bone)—bent or crooked appearance of limb; blue, pale, or purplish appearance of limb; inability of limb to bear weight; severe pain; bones sticking out of the skin (see **Fractures (Broken Bones) and Sprains,** page 129)

3. Wash the wound.

a. If the bleeding can be stopped, wash the wound vigorously with large amounts of soap and water. (Figure 1)

b. If the bleeding restarts after washing the wound, control it again.

4. Cover the wound with a dressing.

a. Use sterile gauze or a clean cloth to make a dressing.

b. Tape the dressing firmly in place or wrap strips of cloth around the dressing. (Figure 2) You should still be able to feel a pulse beneath the dressing. Loosen the dressing slightly if the nail beds of the wounded extremity become blue, the extremity is very cool, or you cannot feel a pulse at a point beyond the wound, away from the center of the body.

5. Observe the animal.

If the Child Was Bitten By a Pet Dog or Cat

a. Find out the animal's immunization date. If possible, check this information by locating the animal's health records or by calling its veterinarian. Do not check its collar as you might be bitten.

b. If the animal's immunization against rabies is not up-to-date, observe the animal for rabies for the next two weeks and notify the child's doctor immediately. If the animal does have rabies, it will be very sick. Symptoms include insatiable thirst, foaming at the mouth, excessive salivation, and possible abnormal behavior (such as aggressiveness). If such symptoms exist, call your county health department and the animal's veterinarian.

Figure 1

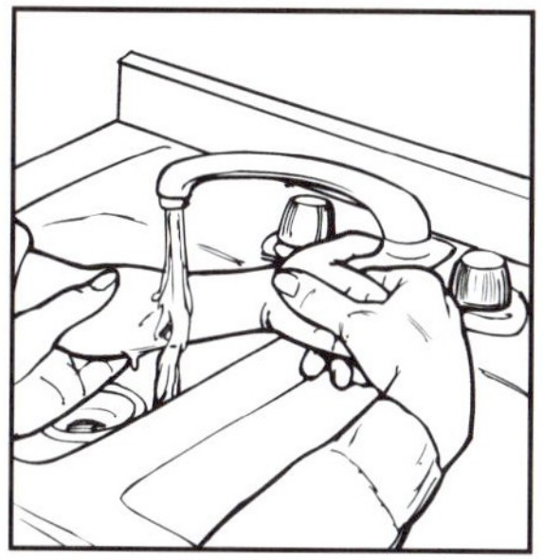

Figure 2

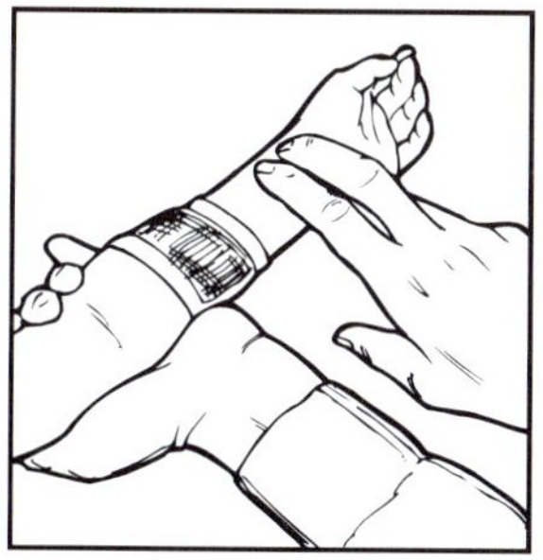

If the Child Was Bitten By a Stray or Wild Animal

a. Notify the child's doctor immediately.
b. Confine the animal, if possible.
c. Contact your county health department; they will have the animal confined and observed for rabies for the next two weeks.
d. If the animal cannot be found or identified, the child may have to receive a series of rabies vaccinations to prevent the onset of rabies.

When to See a Doctor

Take the child to a medical facility if any of the following occur:

1. The skin is broken.
2. Bleeding cannot be controlled within 10 minutes. (**Call 911 or the rescue squad** for a large amount of blood or rapid bleeding, and treat for shock. See **Shock,** page 169.)
3. The bite was caused by an animal that might have rabies (a pet dog or cat whose immunization against rabies is not up-to-date, or a wild or stray animal).

Be prepared to tell the doctor the date of the child's last tetanus shot, if possible. A tetanus shot will not be necessary after a human bite because the organism that causes tetanus is not found in the human mouth.

Safety Highlights

Do

- **Do** watch the child for at least 1 hour following the bite or sting.
- **Do** consult the doctor before using any medications, such as antihistamines.
- **Do** act in a calm manner to prevent anxiety in the child.
- **Do** request a prescription for an insect-sting kit (epinephrine injection) if the child has a history of bee-sting allergies. Learn when and how to use it.

Don't

- **Don't** use tweezers to remove a honeybee stinger from the skin; doing so may squeeze more venom into the child. Instead, use the edge of a razor, knife, or fingernail to scrape the stinger off sideways.
- **Don't** delay treatment for a child showing signs of a severe allergic reaction to an insect bite or sting. **Call 911 or the rescue squad** as soon as symp toms appear. While waiting for medical personnel to arrive, observe the child for breathing difficulty or a change in level of consciousness.

Immediate Action

Check for signs of a reaction to the insect bite or sting. There are two basic kinds of reactions:

Local Reaction There is severe pain and swelling at the site, and the site may be warm and/or reddened. See **Home Treatment,** page 61.

Systemic Reaction This is an allergic reaction affecting many systems of the body. It may become life threatening.

There are three types of systemic reactions:

- *Hives or skin rash*—There are reddened, patchy, itchy areas that may be flat or raised. This indicates that the child is sensitive to that particular insect; future stings or bites could cause a more serious reaction.

- *Asthma attack*—Breathing becomes difficult; there is wheezing, in which "whistling" noises can be heard when the child breathes in and/or out; the child is very anxious and can only concentrate on breathing; the child breathes in deeply, but rapidly (0–1 year—more than sixty times per minute; 1 year and older—more than forty times per minute); the child uses the shoulder and abdominal muscles to breathe, pulling the chest in deeply; and the child's lips, gums, and nails may become pale or bluish. Such an attack is a result of a swelling and narrowing of the air passages.
- *Severe allergic reaction*—There may be facial swelling, nausea, abdominal cramps, muscle cramps, sweating, severe breathing difficulty, fainting, seizure, unconsciousness, or shock.

  NOTE: *A severe allergic reaction is more likely in a child who has hay fever, asthma, or other allergies. Bites from black widow or brown recluse spiders, from scorpions, and from tarantulas also cause these symptoms.*

Observe the appropriate following instructions depending on the type of systemic reaction to the insect bite or sting.

Hives or Skin Rash

1. Observe the child.

Observe him for 1–2 hours after the bite or sting, watching for breathing difficulty, facial swelling, nausea, abdominal cramps, muscle cramps, sweating, or fainting. (Figure 1) See instructions for **Severe Allergic Reaction,** below, if these signs occur.

Figure 1

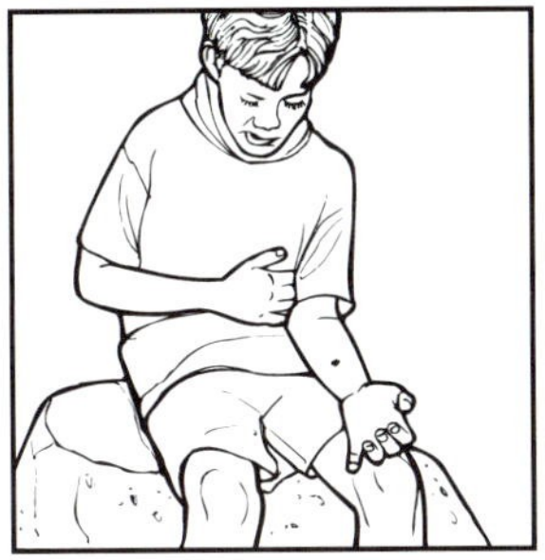

2. If the symptoms do not appear to be a severe allergic reaction,

carry out the instructions indicated in **Home Treatment,** page 61. If rash or hives persist, contact the child's doctor.

Asthma Attack

Treat for asthma as directed in **Breathing Difficulty—Asthma,** page 77. Once asthma is under control, treat the bite or sting by following the instructions indicated in **Home Treatment,** page 61.

Severe Allergic Reaction

1. Check for and treat the most life-threatening problems now.

Check for signs of unconsciousness, no breathing, no pulse, bleeding, or shock. (Figure 2) See **Life-Threat Checklist,** page 23. **Call 911 or the rescue squad** as recommended in **Life-Threat Checklist.**

Figure 2

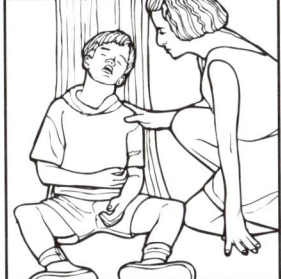

When to See a Doctor

Call 911 or the rescue squad if previously instructed to do so. Otherwise, take the child to see a doctor if any of the following occur:

- severe swelling anywhere on the body, especially the face;
- abdominal pain and/or muscle cramps;
- increasingly difficult breathing;
- nausea;

OR

if the child has a history of allergies to bees, the environment, and so on.

Home Treatment

If the child does not have serious symptoms requiring the attention of a doctor, do the following:

1. Remove the stinger, if present. Do not squeeze the stinger—this will cause it to release more venom. Use the edge of a razor, knife, or fingernail to scrape the stinger off in a sideways fashion.
2. Keep the affected limb down, below the level of the heart.
3. Wash the affected area vigorously with soap and cold water.
4. Apply cold cloths or ice, wrapped in cloth or plastic, to the area.
5. Apply calamine lotion or a paste of baking soda and water to relieve the itching.

Safety Highlights

Do

- **Do** wash the area around the wound as well as the wound itself.
- **Do** feel for a pulse near the wound after you have applied a bandage. It might be necessary to check for the pulse through the bandage layers.
- **Do** press gently on a head wound.

Don't

- **Don't** apply direct pressure on a wound if a fracture (broken bone) is suspected. Signs of a fracture are outlined in **Fractures (Broken Bones) and Sprains,** Step 3, page 130.
- **Don't** apply a bandage so tightly that the area past the bandage turns pale, blue, cold, or numb.
- **Don't** use iodine, merbromin (for example, Mercurochrome®), or other antiseptics without first checking with the doctor.

Immediate Action

1. Look at the surroundings and the general appearance of the child.

(Take a few seconds.)

Was there a severe fall or a forceful blow to the injured area, or was any part of the child's body severely twisted? Is there an obvious broken bone (for example, a deformed limb or a bone sticking out of the skin)? (Figure 1)

Figure 1

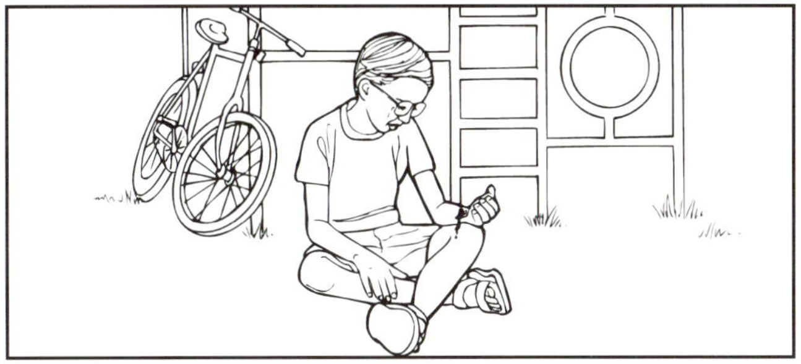

b. While waiting for medical personnel to arrive, press down on the nearest pressure point. See **If Bleeding Cannot Be Immediately Controlled,** pages 66–69.

2. Secure the dressing.

If the bleeding is controlled, hold the dressing (the gauze or cloth on the wound) in place with tape or wrap strips of cloth around it to secure it. You should be able to feel a pulse beneath the dressing. Loosen the dressing slightly if the nail beds of the wounded extremity become blue, the extremity is very cool, or you cannot feel a pulse at a point beyond the wound, away from the center of the body. (Figure 4)

Figure 4

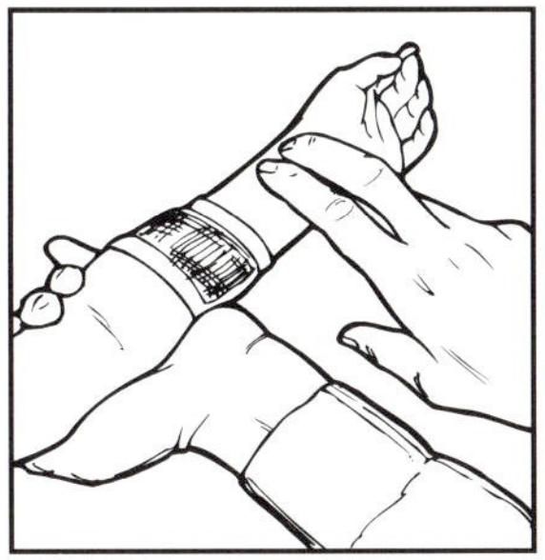

3. Treat for shock.

See **Shock,** page 169.

If a Fracture Is Suspected

Signs of a fracture are outlined on page 130.

1. Do not move the limb.

Leave the limb in the same position in which it was found.

2. Have someone call 911 or the rescue squad.

3. Stop the flow of blood.

Do not press on the wound. Instead, use the pressure point nearest to the wound, located between the heart and the wound, to control bleeding. See **If Bleeding Cannot Be Immediately Controlled,** pages 66–69.

4. Treat for shock.

See **Shock,** page 169.

5. Splint the injured area so it cannot move.

See **Fractures (Broken Bones) and Sprains,** page 132, for splinting techniques.

If Bleeding Cannot Be Immediately Controlled: Arm or Leg Wounds

If bleeding cannot be immediately controlled, use pressure points.

1. If no fracture is suspected, apply direct pressure to the wound.

Continue to press firmly on the wound with sterile gauze or a clean cloth.

2. Keep the injured limb higher than the heart.

NOTE: *Do not move the limb if it causes pain to do so or if a fracture is suspected.*

3. Press firmly on a pressure point.

Pressure points are used to press an artery against a bone to stop bleeding. Follow these steps:

a. Continue to apply direct pressure to the wound with one hand. With the other hand, find the pressure point nearest to the wound, located between the wound and the heart. (Figure 5)

b. Place your thumb on the outside of the injured limb and your fingers on the inside, over the pressure point. (Figure 6) If using a pressure point located in

Figure 5

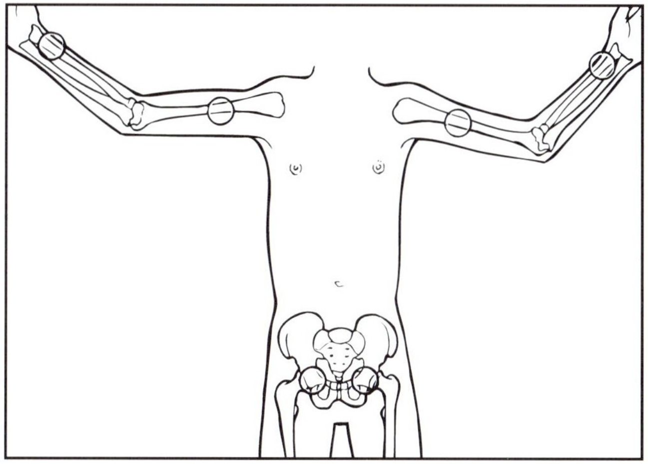

Figure 6

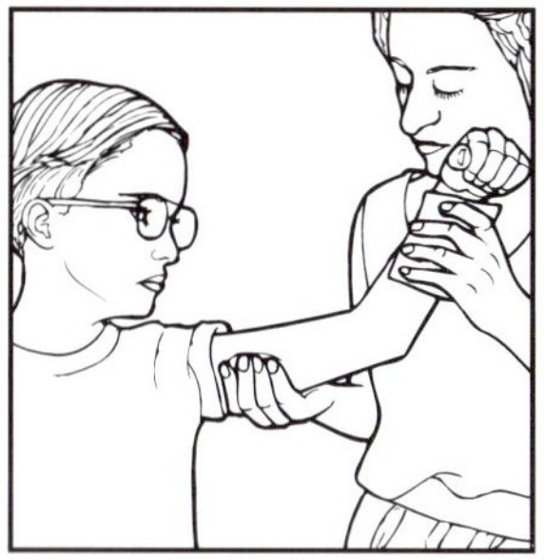

the groin, place your hand flatly over the area of the pressure point and press downward, toward the bone. (Figure 7)

c. Press firmly with the *flat, inside* surface of your fingers, not your fingertips. Press against the bone until the bleeding stops. (Figure 8)

4. If bleeding is still not controlled, call 911 or the rescue squad, if you have not already done so.

Continue to apply pressure to the pressure point and the wound (if no fracture is suspected) while awaiting medical help.

If bleeding is controlled,

a. Release pressure gradually from the pressure point while continuing to press on the wound (if no fracture is suspected).

b. Apply tape or tie strips of cloth around the cloth that is on the wound, to hold the dressing in place. Loosen the dressing slightly if the nail beds of the wounded extremity become blue, the extremity is very cool, or you cannot feel a pulse at a point beyond the wound, away from the center of the body. (Figure 9)

5. Treat for shock.

See **Shock,** page 169.

Figure 7

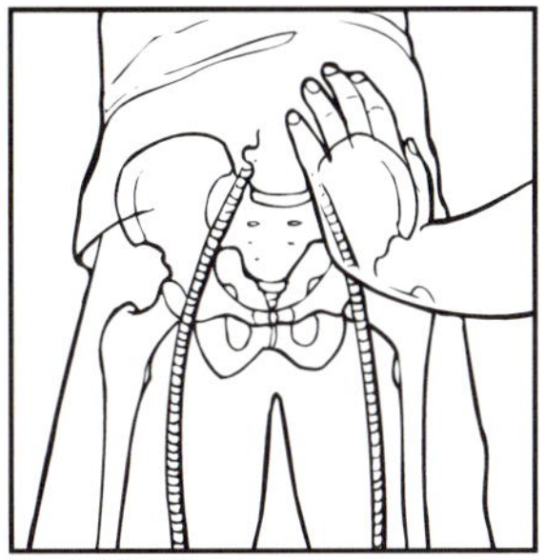

Figure 8

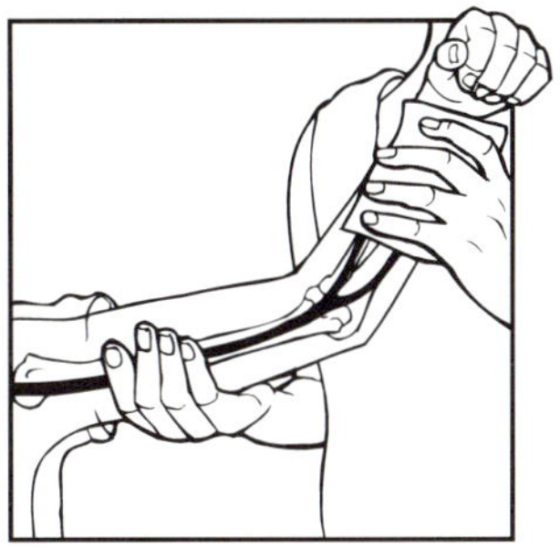

Figure 9

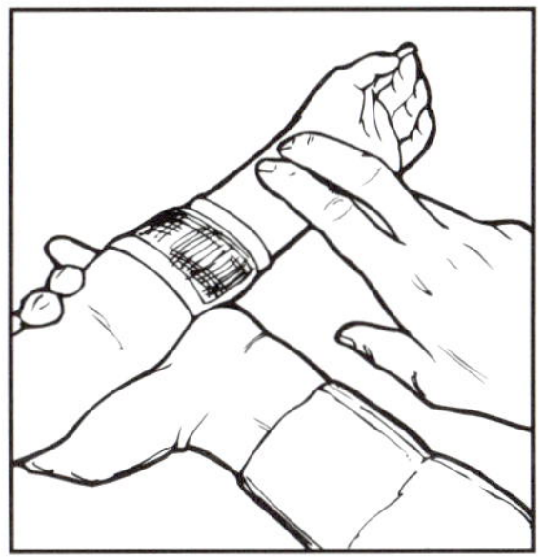

When to See a Doctor

Call 911 or the rescue squad if previously instructed to do so. Otherwise, contact the child's doctor if any of the following occur:

- The cut is deeper than just the skin layers (you may see white fat through the cut).
- You cannot close the wound when you try to bring the edges together.
- The cut is on the face, chest, abdomen, or back (unless very small or shallow).
- There is numbness, tingling, or weakness of an injured limb.
- Foreign objects in the wound cannot be removed.
- A fracture is suspected. See **Fractures (Broken Bones) and Sprains,** page 129.
- The child has not had a tetanus shot within five years and the cut was caused by a dirty or rusty object, or the wound is very dirty.

Home Treatment

A doctor may not be needed for minor cuts. Apply home treatment as follows:

1. Wash the wound well with soap and water.
2. Check for dirt, glass, or other foreign objects in the wound. Remove them gently with a sterile needle or tweezers. (Sterilize the tweezers by boiling them in water for 20 minutes or by holding them over a flame.)
3. Cover the wound with a clean dressing (gauze). Change the dressing daily and if it becomes soiled or wet.
4. Check the wound daily for signs of infection. If infected, the wound may be red, hot, tender, or swollen or have pus (thick, yellow or green drainage); the child may have a fever. If an infection is present, call the child's doctor to have the wound examined.

The following is background information. You are not expected to diagnose the child, but information regarding the causes of breathing difficulty is often helpful.

Children's airways are very small and narrow. They can become swollen and thus narrower as a result of viruses, bacteria, emotional upset, or allergies. They also can be easily blocked by a foreign object. Some of the most common causes of breathing difficulty in children are the following:

Croup Croup is usually caused by a virus. Noisy breathing, hoarseness, and a barking cough are the most common signs. The child also may be breathing at an abnormally rapid rate, be pulling in her chest and/or stomach muscles extremely deeply when she breathes, be gasping for air, and she may be getting agitated or extremely anxious. Croup is worse at night. It is most common in children under 4 years old.

Epiglottitis Epiglottitis is a severe infection of the throat, causing such great swelling of the tissue above the windpipe that it is very difficult for the child to breathe. The most common sign is an extreme difficulty swallowing. The child usually will be breathing noisily and at an abnormally rapid rate, pulling in her chest and/or stomach muscles extremely deeply when she breathes, and she may be getting anxious. The child might gasp for air, and lips, gums, and/or nails may be pale or bluish in color. A fever over 102°F is also common. This infection requires immediate medical attention. It is most common in children over 3 years old.

Pneumonia Pneumonia is an infection of the lungs, usually following a cold. It also may occur if a foreign substance is inhaled into the lungs. The most common signs are abnormally rapid breathing, a deep pulling-in of chest and/or stomach muscles, and anxiety. If the pneumonia is severe, lips, gums, and nails may turn pale or bluish in color. A fever may also be present. Pneumonia requires immediate medical attention.

Asthma, or Reactive Airway Disease With asthma, the small airways in the lungs become very narrow, and extra mucus is produced. The child has to work harder to force the air out of the lungs and also feels as if not enough air is getting in. Asthma may be caused by an allergy to pollen, dust, grass, animal hair, or some foods; an infection in the airways; a change in weather; exercise; smoke; continuous high-level activity; or emotional upset. The most common symptom is wheezing. Other common signs include abnormally rapid breathing, a pulling-in of chest and/or stomach muscles, and anxiety. The child may have a congested cough and be gasping for air. If the asthma is severe, lips, gums, and nails may be pale or bluish in color. A family usually learns to treat asthma attacks at home, but if treatment is unsuccessful, immediate medical attention is required.

Foreign body in airway An object may partially block the airway, causing difficulty in breathing. This may result in wheezing or high-pitched noises, and it may be mistaken for asthma. The most common sign is violent coughing. A foreign body should be suspected if the event occurred suddenly in an infant or small child known to put "everything" in his or her mouth. See **Choking:** 0–1 year, page 91; 1+ years, page 103.

- Gasping for air.
- Wheezing, or making whistling noises as he breathes in and/or out.
- Experiencing lips, gums, or nails that are pale or a bluish color.

2. Decide whether to seek medical assistance.

a. **Call 911 or rescue squad** if the child has signs of breathing difficulty *and*

- He is gasping for air, or
- His lips, gums, or nails are pale or a bluish color.

b. Take the child to a medical facility immediately if he has any of the following signs:

- Pulling in his chest and/or stomach muscles so deeply that you can see his ribs.
- Breathing much more rapidly than usual (0–1 year—more than sixty times per minute; 1+ years—more than forty times per minute).
- Looking very anxious, with trouble breathing, or he tells you he is having trouble breathing.
- Wheezing, or making whistling noises as he breathes in and/or out. (This may be an asthma attack. See **Asthma,** page 77.)
- Difficulty swallowing, which is causing drooling, and breathing with his mouth wide open and his chin jutting forward. Keep the child sitting in an upright position.

c. Call the child's doctor if the child has either of the following signs:

- A congested cough, causing a "rattling" feeling when you feel his chest or back.
- A fever with signs of a cold, such as cough and/or congestion.

d. Follow **Home Treatment,** page 75, if the child has either of the following signs:

- A cough resembling the barking of a seal but no signs of severe breathing difficulty. The problem may be croup, as described on page 71.
- Signs of a cold, such as nasal congestion, but no fever.

3. Maximize the child's breathing ability.

Until medical help arrives, or on the way to a medical facility,

a. Sit the child in an upright position. If you suspect a back or neck injury, leave the child flat.

b. Position the child so that the head is not over-extended in either a forward or backward position, obstructing the airway.

c. Do not give the child anything to drink.

d. If the child is nasally congested, help clear her nose. (Use a bulb syringe or aspirator for an infant or toddler.)

4. Reduce the child's anxiety.

a. Speak and act in a calm manner. Anxiety can cause the child's airways to narrow.

b. Keep the child calm and quiet. Have the child look at you and breathe as slowly and deeply as she can. Breathe with the child for as long as she will cooperate, inhaling deeply through the nose, holding the breath, and breathing out through pursed lips as if blowing out candles. (Figure 1)

c. Keep the child's environment quiet.

d. Use soothing talk or gestures to relax the child. Alternate soothing talk with slow breathing techniques to hold the child's interest.

e. Allow the child to hold a security object (such as a

Figure 1

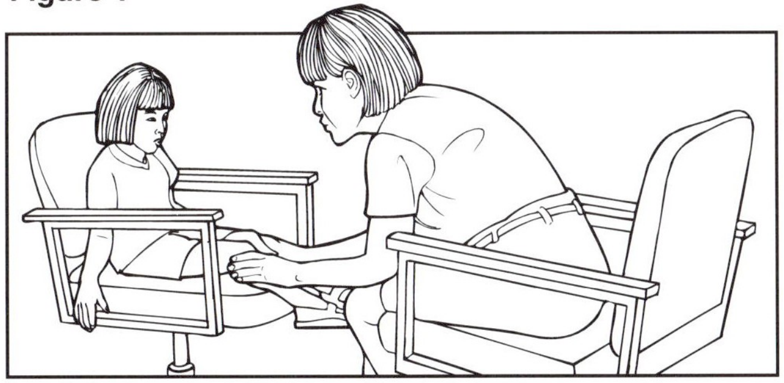

When to See a Doctor

Call 911 or the rescue squad if previously instructed to do so. Or, take the child to a medical facility immediately as recommended on page 73. Otherwise, take the child to see a doctor if the child is under 6 months old and/or any of the following occur:

- Efforts to relieve breathing difficulty are not helpful.
- The child's condition worsens.
- The child has a fever over 101°F with breathing difficulty.

Home Treatment

If the child has a cough that sounds like a barking seal but is not suffering as severely as previously described, provide humidity:

1. Fill the bathroom with steam from a hot shower.
2. Have the child breathe in the steam for 20 minutes. (Do not have the child sit on the floor; steam rises. Do not hold her too close to the water; the steam or splashing water may burn the skin.) (Figure 2)
3. If no relief occurs within 20 minutes, take the child outside to breathe fresh air.
4. If the child is breathing easier and not coughing as much, put her in bed with a vaporizer placed a few feet away (out of reach of a young child). (Figure 3)
5. If the child's condition worsens or if there is no relief, call the doctor.

If the child has signs of a cold, with congestion and mild breathing difficulty, do the following:

1. Increase the child's fluid intake. Clear liquids (water, juice, gelatin) are best to make the mucus less thick.

Figure 2

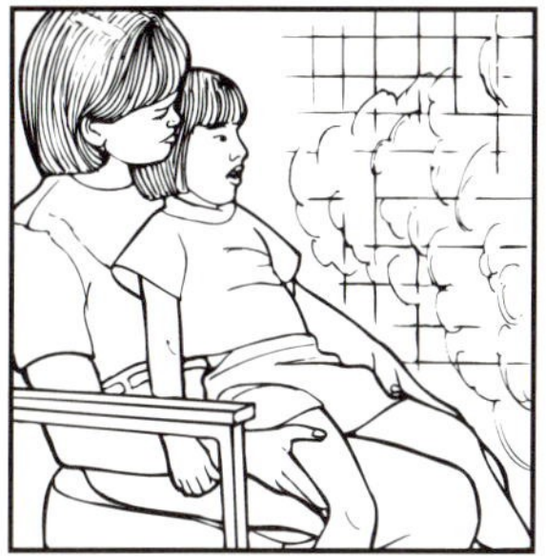

Figure 3

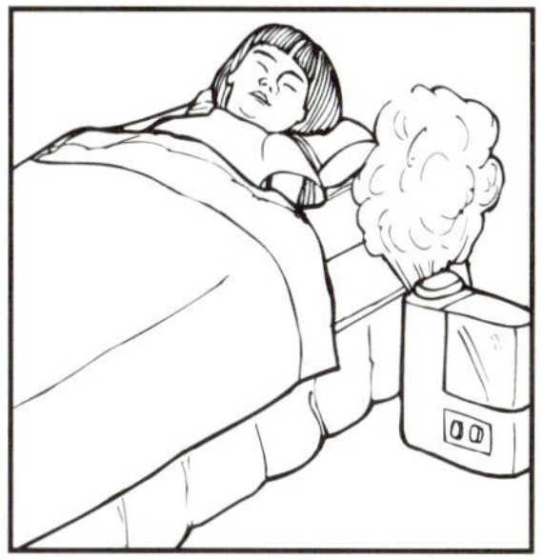

Safety Highlights

Do

- **Do** act calmly to prevent anxiety and greater breathing difficulty for the child.
- **Do** sit the child in an upright position to ease breathing.
- **Do** consider the possibility of a foreign object in the airway if the attack came on suddenly and the child was eating or normally puts "everything" in his or her mouth, and if the child cannot cry or speak.

Don't

- **Don't** take time to provide humidity with a vaporizer or shower; it will not help an asthma attack.
- **Don't** give the child his or her asthma medication if you are not the child's parent or legal guardian. Contact the child's parent or legal guardian first. If unavailable, contact the child's doctor.

Immediate Action

1. Check for signs and symptoms of asthma.

The child is

- Breathing much more rapidly than usual (1+ years—more than forty times per minute; 0–1 year—more than sixty times per minute; but asthma is uncommon in infants). Calm the child, then count the breathing rate.
- Wheezing, or making whistling noises as she breathes in and/or out.
- Experiencing a harsh or congested cough. (This may not happen.)
- Looking anxious, or she tells you she is having trouble breathing.

- Experiencing a rapid heart rate or pulse (1+ years—more than 130 beats per minute; 0–1 year—more than 160 beats per minute). See **How to Check a Child's Vital Signs,** page 13.
- Pulling in her chest and/or stomach muscles so deeply that you can see her ribs much more easily than usual.
- Experiencing lips, gums, or nails that are pale or a bluish color.

NOTE: *All symptoms may not be present. Asthma may be mild and not affect the child very much, or it may be severe, causing great difficulty in breathing.*

2. Follow the appropriate instructions as follows.

- If the child has been treated for asthma in the past, proceed to **If the Child Has Previously Been Treated for Asthma,** page 80.
- Otherwise, follow instructions for **If the Child Has Not Been Treated for Asthma Before,** below.

If the Child Has Not Been Treated for Asthma Before

1. Seek medical assistance.

a. Call 911 or the rescue squad if:

- The child is having severe breathing difficulty and her lips, gums, and nails are pale or a bluish color, or
- The child becomes unconscious after having breathing difficulty.

b. Take the child to a medical facility immediately if the child has never been treated for asthma before but has any of the asthma symptoms listed in Step 1,

2. Maximize the child's breathing ability.

While awaiting medical help or on the way to a medical facility,

a. Sit the child in an upright position. Help the child choose a comfortable position; many children prefer to lean foward, supporting their weight on a table or chair. (Figure 1)

b. Do not give the child anything to drink.

3. Reduce the child's anxiety.

a. Speak and act in a calm manner. Anxiety can cause the child's airways to narrow.

b. Keep the child calm and quiet. Use slow-breathing techniques with the child, inhaling deeply through the nose, holding the breath, and breathing out through pursed lips as if blowing out candles. Have the child look at you and breathe as slowly and deeply as possible. Breathe with the child for as long as she will cooperate. (Figure 2)

c. Keep the child's environment quiet.

d. Use soothing talk or gestures to relax the child. Alternate soothing talk with slow-breathing techniques to hold the child's interest.

e. Allow the child to hold a security object (such as a favorite stuffed animal, blanket, or doll).

Figure 1

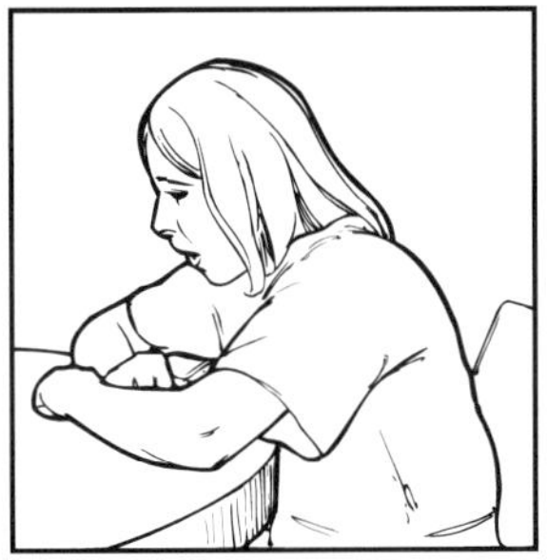

Figure 2

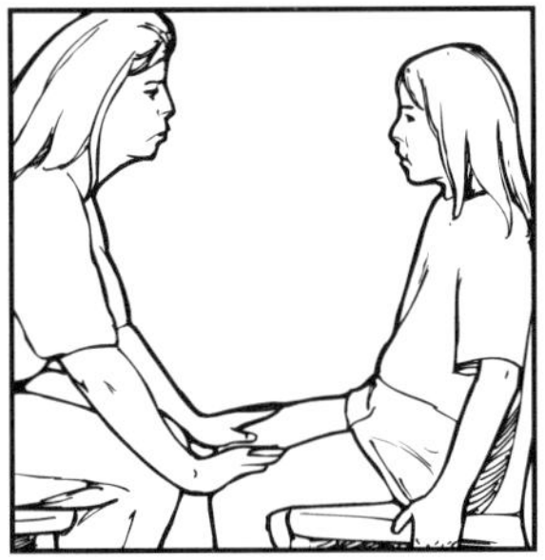

d. Use soothing talk or gestures to relax the child. Alternate soothing talk with slow-breathing techniques to hold the child's interest.

e. Allow the child to hold a security object (such as a favorite stuffed animal, blanket, or doll).

4. Seek medical attention.

Call the child's doctor or take her to the nearest medical facility if the asthma medication has not helped the child breathe easier within 2 hours.

When to See a Doctor

Call 911 or the rescue squad if previously instructed to do so. Otherwise, take the child to see a doctor if the child has never been treated for asthma before and/or:

- Efforts to relieve breathing difficulty are not helpful.
- The child's condition worsens.

Home Treatment

If breathing difficulty has been relieved, do the following:

1. Give the child her prescribed asthma medication as ordered by the doctor, if you are the child's parent or legal guardian.
2. Reduce the child's exposure to allergens; these are things in her environment to which she is very sensitive, such as dust, pollen, animal hair, strong odors (perfume, room deodorizers, and so on), and smoke. Allergens may trigger an asthma attack. If you do not know which allergens the child is sensitive to, consult with the child's doctor. You may be referred to an allergist for allergy testing.

There are different severities of burns and different approaches to treating each. In the event of a medical emergency involving burns, it is helpful to understand the distinctions between the three types of burns:

First degree The skin is smooth, red, and painful, but *not* broken. (Sunburn is an example.)

Second degree Several layers of skin may have been burned; the area is red or purplish; blisters may appear; there is pain and some swelling.

Third degree The skin has a white or grayish appearance; all skin layers have been destroyed. The tissue under the skin can be seen; there is no pain because nerve endings have been destroyed.

Safety Highlights

Do

- **Do** check the burned area for numbness during cold application. If the area is numb, stop cold application to prevent frostbite.
- **Do** use sterile gauze dressings as soon as they are available.
- **Do** check with the doctor before using an antibiotic ointment.

Don't

- **Don't** burst any blisters.
- **Don't** put pressure on the burned area.
- **Don't** touch a burn where the skin has been broken—bacteria on your fingers may cause an infection.
- **Don't** apply any anesthetic sprays, creams, butter, or petroleum jelly—they may make the burn worse, slow healing, and increase the chance of infection.
- **Don't** remove clothing that is stuck to the burn.
- **Don't** apply ice to a burn.
- **Don't** immerse a large burned area in cold water for more than 10 minutes—it may lower the child's body temperature too much.

First- and Second-Degree Burns

Follow the instructions below if *first-degree* burns are present

OR

if *second-degree* burns are present in which:

- the skin is not broken.
- the burn is not on the face, hands, feet, or genitals.

1. Protect the burned area.

a. After applying cold cloths, as indicated above in **Immediate Action,** Step 1, blot the area dry with sterile gauze.

b. Apply a clean dressing over the burned area. Use sterile gauze or a clean cloth. Keep the dressing in place with

- A gauze bandage or strips of cloth. When wrapping, start at the bottom of the dressing and gently wrap up, toward the heart. (Figures 4, 5) Place a piece of tape on the bandage to prevent it from unwinding, or make a lengthwise cut in the end of the bandage, approximately six to eight inches long, and tie the ends around the wrapped area to secure it. Your finger should easily slip under the dressing, allowing room for swelling. The dressing must not be tight.
- Tape, if the burn is not on a limb. The dressing should cover an area larger than the burn so the tape can be applied to healthy skin.

Figure 4

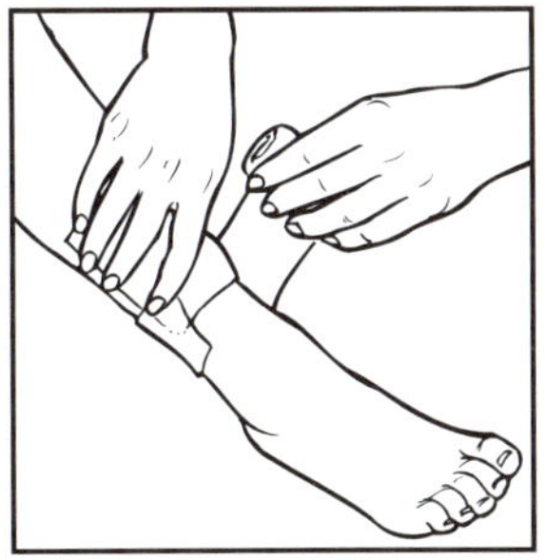

Figure 5

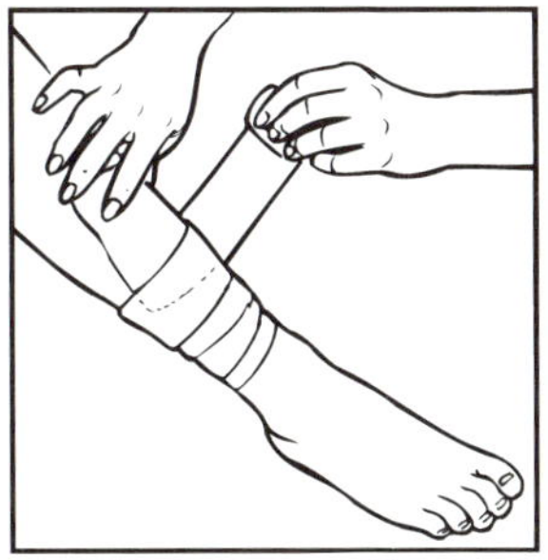

2. Reduce the swelling.

a. If the burn is on an arm or a leg, raise it higher than the heart.

b. Reapply cold cloths, wrapped in plastic. Place them over the dressing. (Figure 6) Check every 10 minutes for numbness, and remove the cloths when the pain decreases or if the area becomes numb.

Figure 6

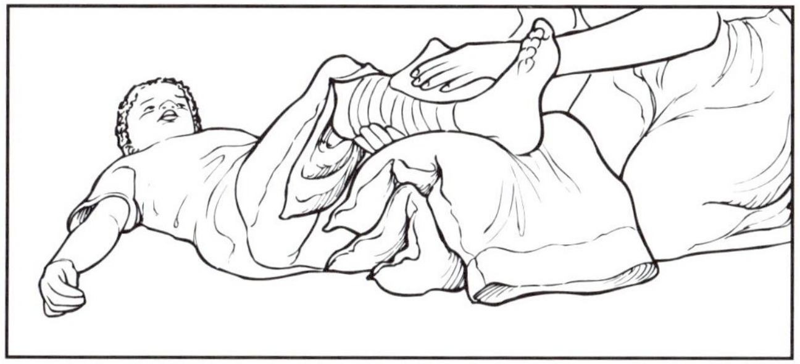

3. Reduce the pain.

a. Application of cold cloths, as described in Step 2, should help relieve pain.

b. Give the child acetaminophen, a nonaspirin pain reliever. (Do not medicate the child if you are not the child's parent or legal guardian. Contact the parents or the child's doctor first.) If you do give medication, follow the dosage recommended on the label or in the Acetaminophen Dosage Chart shown here.

4. See When to See a Doctor and Home Treatment, pages 89 and 90.

Acetaminophen Dosage Chart

Age	Weight (in pounds)	80 milligram drops, 0.8 milliliters per dropperful (dppr.)	160 milligram elixir, 5 milliliters per teaspoon	80 milligram chewable tablets	160 milligram junior-strength tablets
0–3 mo.	6–11 lb.	½ dppr. (0.4 ml)	—	—	—
4–11 mo.	12–17 lb.	1 dppr. (0.8 ml)	½ teaspoon	1 tablet	—
12–23 mo.	18–23 lb.	1½ dppr. (1.2 ml)	¾ teaspoon	1½ tablets	—
2–3 yr.	24–35 lb.	2 dppr. (1.6 ml)	1 teaspoon	2 tablets	—
4–5 yr.	36–47 lb.	—	1½ teaspoons	3 tablets	—
6–8 yr.	48–59 lb.	—	2 teaspoons	4 tablets	2 tablets
9–10 yr.	60–71 lb.	—	2½ teaspoons	5 tablets	2½ tablets
11 yr.	72–95 lb.	—	3 teaspoons	6 tablets	3 tablets
12–14 yr.	96 lb. and over	—	—	—	4 tablets

Severe Second- and Third-Degree Burns

Follow the instructions below if *second-degree* burns are present in which:

- the skin is broken.
- the involved area is greater than the size of the child's hand.
- the face, hands, feet, or genitals are involved. (Burns may result in cosmetic problems or loss of function.)

OR

if signs of a *third-degree* burn are present.

1. Seek medical assistance.

Call 911 or the rescue squad if:

- The burn is very severe and you think it may be a third-degree burn.
- The child is having difficulty breathing. (Smoke inhalation or burns involving the face may cause the airways to swell, making breathing difficult.) See **Breathing Difficulty—General,** page 71.
- The child becomes unconscious. See **Life-Threat Checklist,** page 23, immediately.
- The child shows signs of shock. See **Shock,** page 169.

While awaiting medical help, follow Steps 2–6. If symptoms are not as severe as those noted above, follow Steps 2–6 and call the child's doctor.

2. Protect the burned area.

a. Cut off any clothing around the burn, but do not remove clothing that is stuck to the burn. (Figure 7)

Figure 7

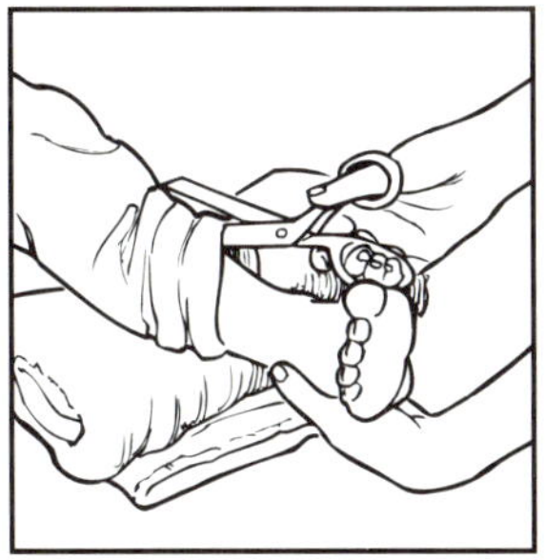

6. Prevent dehydration.

If medical help does not arrive or you cannot reach medical assistance within 1 hour, and the child is awake, conscious, not vomiting, and not having trouble breathing, provide fluids. (Figure 12)

a. Add 1 level teaspoon of salt and $\frac{1}{2}$ level teaspoon of baking soda to 1 quart (32 ounces) of warm water. Give this solution to the child as follows:

- Infant (under 1 year): 1 ounce
- Small child (1–8 years): 2 ounces
- Older child (8+ years): 4 ounces

b. Stop giving the fluid if the child vomits.

c. Give water instead of the salt solution, if that is all you have. (Burns can cause a large fluid loss, which may cause the child to go into shock.)

Figure 12

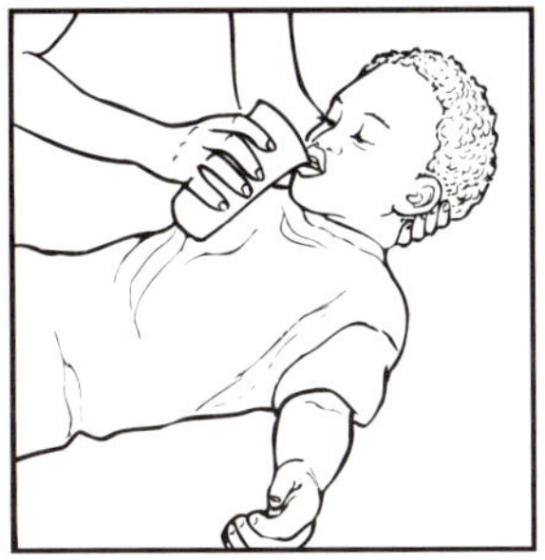

When to See a Doctor

Call 911 or rescue squad if previously instructed to do so. After the initial action is taken, take the child to see a doctor if any of the following apply:

- The burn covers an area larger than the size of the child's hand.
- The burn is on the face, hands, feet, or genitals.
- The skin has been broken.
- The burned area remains extremely painful for more than 48 hours.
- Signs of an infection develop—there is pus (thick, yellowish or greenish drainage); the area around the burn is red, swollen, hard, and painful when touched; or fever develops.

Home Treatment

If the child's burn is not as serious as described above, do the following:

1. If a cloth dressing was applied to the burn, replace it with a sterile gauze dressing as soon as one is available. (A dressing is not needed for sunburns.) Keep the dressing clean and dry.
2. Change the dressing once daily and if it becomes soiled or wet. Inspect the burn for signs of infection during dressing changes and if the child develops a fever.
3. If blisters burst, use a nonstick type of dressing; use tape to hold it in place.
4. Apply antibiotic ointments only as ordered by the child's doctor.
5. Apply cool cloths to a sunburn, and over the dressing for other burns, for pain relief. Cover the dressing with plastic first.

Safety Highlights

Do

- **Do** support the infant's head when repositioning him or her for back blows or chest thrusts.
- **Do** place your fingertips along the infant's breast-bone correctly for chest thrusts.

Don't

- **Don't** interfere while the infant is coughing—allow the infant to cough out the object.
- **Don't** shake the infant to dislodge the object or to make the child breathe.
- **Don't** reach inside the infant's mouth for an object unless it can be seen.
- **Don't** press down on the infant's ribs when delivering chest thrusts.

Immediate Action

If the Choking Infant Is Conscious (Awake)

If the choking infant is unconscious, see **If the Choking Infant Is Unconscious (Not Responsive),** page 95. If the choking infant is conscious, do the following:

1. Check the infant for signs of choking:

- The infant cannot cough or cry.
- The infant can make only high-pitched noises or no noises at all.
- The infant is anxious.

b. Place your next two fingers on the infant's breastbone, next to your ring finger.

c. Raise your ring finger up, off the infant's chest. (Figure 3)

d. Use just the tips of the two remaining fingers to deliver chest thrusts.

NOTE: *You should not be pressing down on the lower tip of the breastbone. (You can feel where it ends.) You may find that you are pressing on the breastbone tip if your hand is large. If so, move your fingers up toward the infant's head slightly, away from the breastbone tip.*

Figure 3

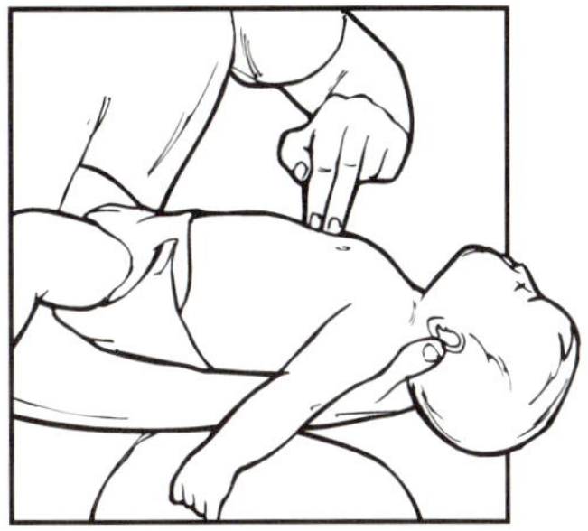

6. Give five chest thrusts.

a. With the tips of two fingers, press directly downward toward the infant's back to a depth of $\frac{1}{2}$ to 1 inch. Use a quick, deliberate motion to try to force out of the windpipe the object that is causing the infant to choke. (Figure 4)

b. Repeat four times, pausing for about 1 second between each thrust.

Figure 4

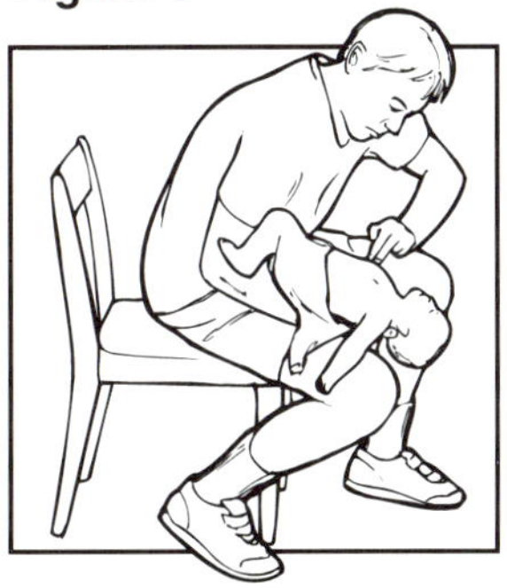

7. Repeat Steps 2–6 three times.

8. Seek medical assistance.

If three cycles of back blows and chest thrusts are unsuccessful in dislodging the object on which the infant is choking, **call 911 or the rescue squad.** Return to the infant.

9. Repeat Steps 2–6 until:

- The object is dislodged. Proceed to Step 10.
- The infant becomes unconscious (limp, not responsive). See **If the Choking Infant Is Unconscious (Not Responsive),** page 95, if this happens.
- Medical help arrives.

10. Check breathing.

If the infant is breathing, see **When to See a Doctor,** page 101.

If the infant is not crying or if you are not sure if the infant is breathing:

a. Position the infant on his back.

b. Open the airway:

   1. Place one hand on the infant's forehead.
   2. Place the fingers of your other hand on the bony part of the lower jaw.
   3. Tilt the infant's head back. The middle of the back of his head should be flat, and the corner of his mouth should be in line with his earlobe.
   4. Keep your hand on the infant's forehead to keep the airway open.

c. Place your ear over the infant's mouth and look at his chest. Look, listen, and feel for a breath for 3–5 seconds. (Figure 5)

d. If the infant is not breathing, see **Rescue Breathing/Cardiopulmonary Resuscitation (CPR),** page 27. If the infant is breathing, see **When to See a Doctor,** page 101.

Figure 5

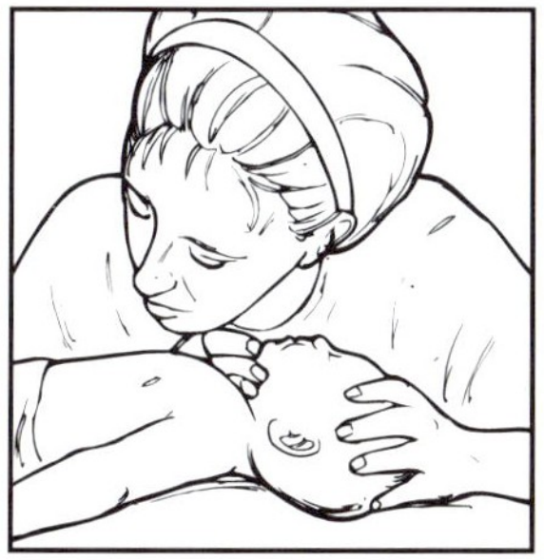

If the Choking Infant Is Unconscious (Not Responsive)

1. Check for signs of unconsciousness:

- There is no response when you gently shake the infant's shoulder. (Figure 6)
- The infant is limp.
- The infant may have a pale, blue, or gray color, and his lips, gums, and nails may be blue.

2. Shout for help.

Have someone **call 911 or the rescue squad,** if you have not already done so. While someone seeks help or if you are alone, follow the steps below.

3. Position the infant face up.

Support the infant's head and neck and turn the infant onto his back. (Figure 7)

4. Open the airway.

a. Place one hand on the infant's forehead.

b. Place the fingers of your other hand on the bony part of the lower jaw.

c. Tilt the infant's head back. The middle of the back of his head should be flat, and the corner of his mouth should be in line with his earlobe. (Figure 8)

d. Keep your hand on the infant's forehead to keep the airway open throughout the next steps.

5. Check breathing.

While holding the airway open, place your ear over the infant's mouth and look at his chest and abdomen. Look, listen, and feel for breath for 3–5 seconds. (Figure 9)

Figure 6

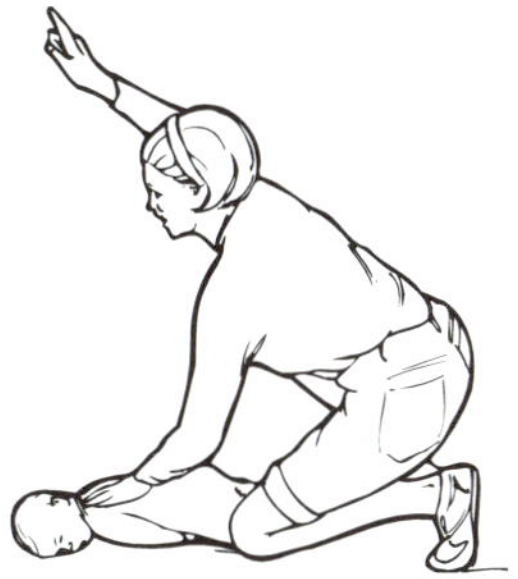

Figure 7

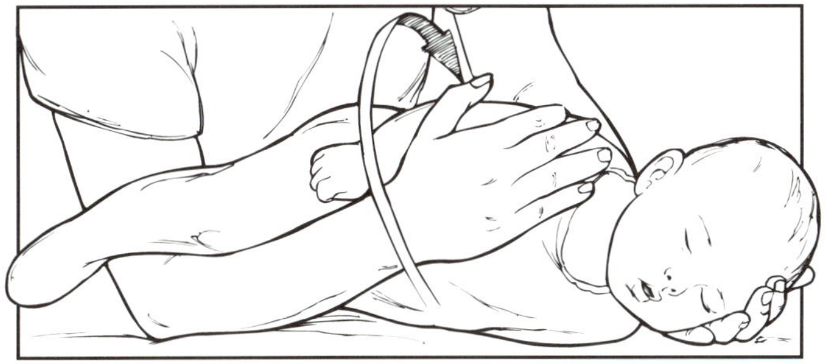

Figure 8

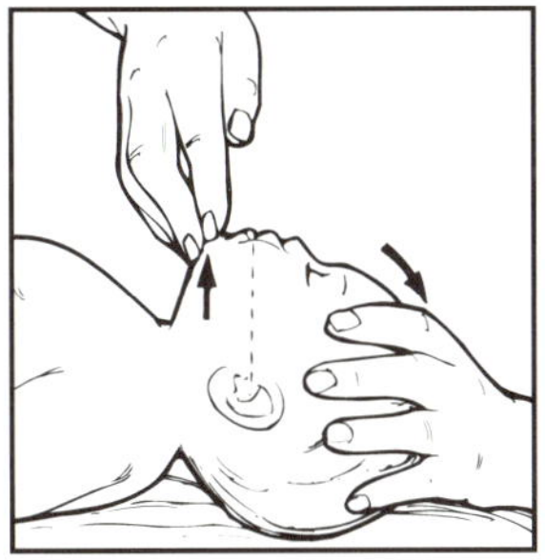

Figure 9

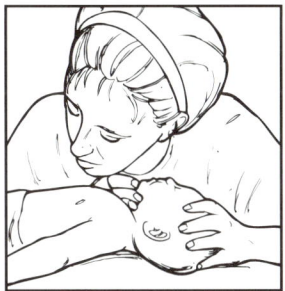

7. Determine if air is entering the infant's lungs.

If air goes in easily and the infant's chest rises, proceed with rescue breathing as instructed in **Rescue Breathing/Cardiopulmonary Resuscitation (CPR),** beginning with Step 7, page 30.

If air does not go in easily and the infant's chest does not rise, the airway remains blocked. Follow Steps 8–16.

8. Position the infant face down.

a. Place the infant face down along the length of your forearm (the infant's jaw should rest in your fingers).

b. Lower your arm—the infant's head should be lower than his feet.

c. Hold the infant against your body or thigh for extra support. Hold his head firmly.

9. Give five back blows.

Using the heel of your free hand, give five forceful back blows, high on the infant's back, between the shoulder blades. (Figure 12)

10. If the object on which the infant is choking has not become dislodged, reposition the infant face up.

a. Sandwich the infant between your arms and turn the infant onto his back, along the length of your forearm.

b. Lower your arm—the infant's head should be lower than his feet. (Figure 13)

Figure 12

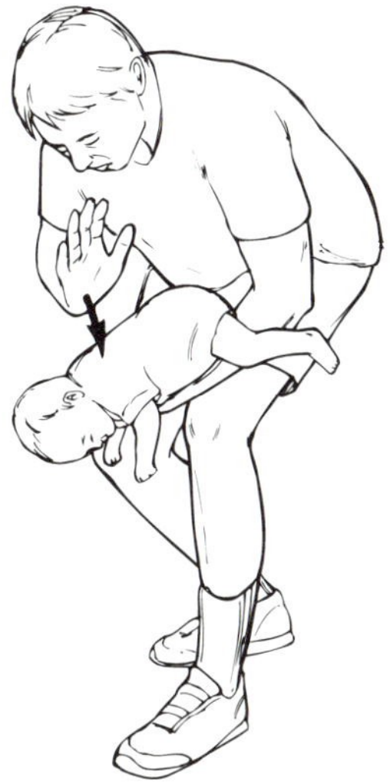

Figure 13

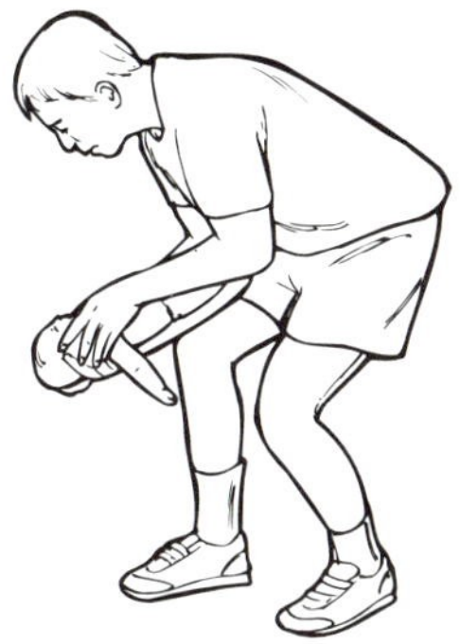

11. Find the correct finger placement for chest thrusts.

a. Place your ring finger on the infant's breastbone at the level of the nipples. Point toward the infant's arm.

b. Place your next two fingers on the infant's breastbone, next to your ring finger.

c. Raise your ring finger up, off the infant's chest. (Figure 14)

d. Use just the tips of the two remaining fingers to deliver chest thrusts.

NOTE: *You should not be pressing down on the lower tip of the breastbone. (You can feel where it ends.) Your may find that you are pressing on the breastbone tip if your hand is large. If so, move your fingers up toward the infant's head slightly, away from the breastbone tip.*

Figure 14

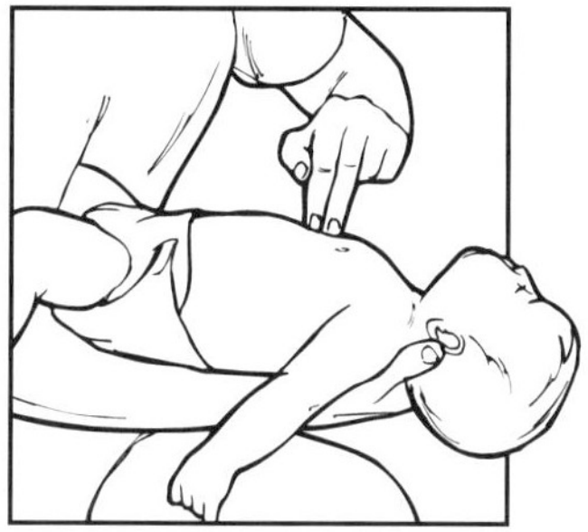

12. Give five chest thrusts.

a. With the tips of two fingers, press directly downward toward the infant's back to a depth of $\frac{1}{2}$ to 1 inch. Use a quick, deliberate motion to try to force out of the windpipe the object that is causing the infant to choke. (Figure 15)

b. Repeat four more times, pausing for about 1 second between each thrust.

Figure 15

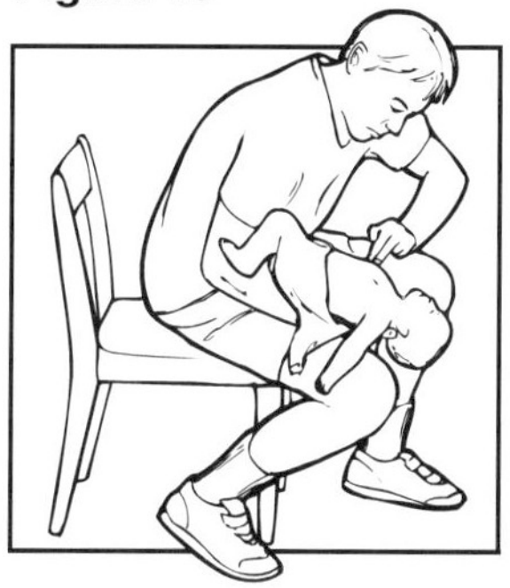

13. Check for the foreign object.

a. Position the infant on his back.

b. Place your thumb on top of the infant's tongue, wrap your fingers under the infant's jaw, and pull the jaw down to open the mouth. Look into the mouth. (Figure 16)

If you see a foreign object: Try to remove it. Use your index finger in a hooked position. Move the finger sideways to sweep the object to the side of the

Figure 16

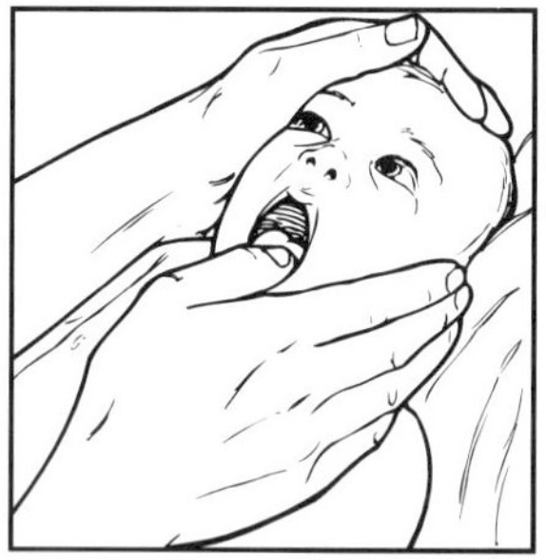

mouth. This will prevent the object from being pushed downward, farther into the throat.

NOTE: *You may have removed only part of the object. Continue to Step 14 to determine airway clearance.*

If you do not see an object: Do not probe into the throat. Proceed to Step 14 instead.

14. Open the airway.

a. Place one hand on the infant's forehead.

b. Place the fingers of your other hand on the bony part of the lower jaw.

c. Tilt the infant's head back. The middle of the back of his head should be flat, and the corner of his mouth should be in line with his earlobe. (Figure 17)

d. Keep your hand on the infant's forehead to keep the airway open throughout the following steps.

Figure 17

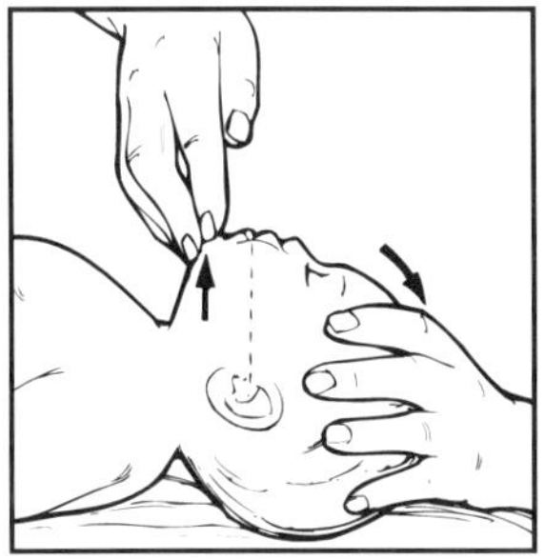

15. Give two rescue breaths.

a. Leaving your hand on the infant's forehead, tightly cover the infant's mouth and nose with your mouth. (Figure 18)

b. Gently blow into the infant's mouth for 1 second.

c. Look at or feel the infant's chest when giving a breath—the chest should rise as the lungs fill with air.

d. If you feel resistance, as if the breath did not go in easily, reposition the infant's head and try again.

Figure 18

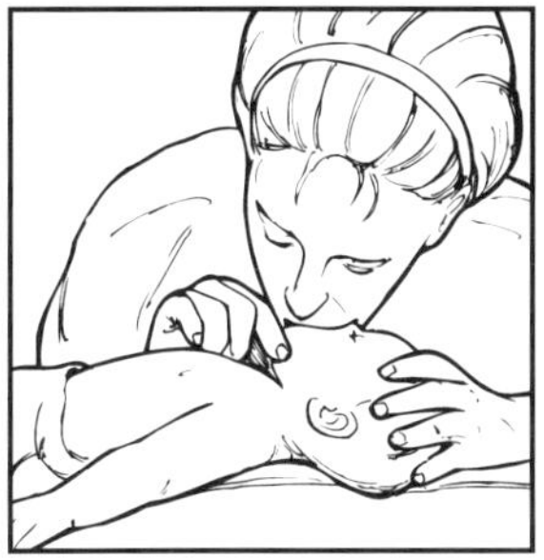

16. Repeat Steps 8–15 three times.

17. Seek medical assistance.

If three cycles of back blows, chest thrusts, and rescue breaths have been unsuccessful, **call 911 or the rescue squad,** if you have not already done so.

When to See a Doctor

After the initial action is taken, take the child to see a doctor if any of the following apply:

- The child's windpipe is cleared of the foreign object and she begins to breathe on her own, but she had been unconscious.
- The child develops a fever and symptoms of a cold within a few days. (Part of the foreign object may have been inhaled into a lung, causing an infection.) Other symptoms to report include cough, fatigue, loss of appetite, and pain in the chest.
- The child has any difficulty breathing.

Home Treatment

Follow-up treatment involves observing the child over the next few days for the symptoms noted above.

Safety Highlights

Do

- **Do** place the heel of your hand on the child's abdomen correctly for abdominal thrusts.
- **Do** adjust the force of abdominal thrusts according to the size of the child.

Don't

- **Don't** interfere while the child is coughing—allow the child to cough out the object.
- **Don't** reach inside the child's mouth for an object unless it can be seen, if the child is under 8 years old.
- **Don't** press down on the child's ribs when delivering abdominal thrusts.

Immediate Action

If the Choking Child Is Conscious (Awake)

If the choking child is unconscious, see **If the Choking Child Is Unconscious (Not Responsive),** page 106. Otherwise, do the following:

1. Check the child for signs of choking:

- The child cannot cough, speak, or cry.
- The child can make only high-pitched noises or no noises at all.
- The child is anxious.
- The child is holding her throat.
- The child responds positively when asked, "Are you choking?"

5. Check for success.

Check for ability to cough, speak, or cry, and for any increase in blueness around the mouth and lips.

a. If the child can cough, do not interfere with her attempts to dislodge the obstruction and regain a regular breathing pattern. If the object is cleared, see **When to See a Doctor,** page 112.

b. If the child still cannot cough or speak, the airway remains obstructed. Proceed to Step 6.

6. Repeat Steps 2–5 three times, as necessary.

7. Seek medical assistance.

If three cycles of abdominal thrusts have been unsuccessful, **call 911 or the rescue squad.** Return to the child.

8. Repeat Steps 2–5 until:

- The object is dislodged. Proceed to Step 9.
- The child becomes unconscious (limp, not responsive). See **If the Choking Child Is Unconscious (Not Responsive),** page 106, if this happens.
- Medical help arrives.

9. Check breathing.

If the child is breathing, see **When to See a Doctor,** page 112.

If the child is not crying or if you are not sure if the child is breathing:

a. Position the child on her back.

b. Open the airway:

1. Place one hand on the child's forehead.
2. Place the fingers of your other hand on the bony part of the chin.
3. Lift the chin and tilt the child's head back. The middle of the back of her head should be flat, and the corner of her mouth should be in line with her earlobe. The neck should not be over-extended or stretched far back. (Figure 3)
4. Keep your hand on the child's forehead to keep the airway open.

c. Place your ear over the child's mouth and look at her chest. Look, listen, and feel for a breath for 3–5 seconds. (Figure 4)

d. If the child is not breathing, see **Rescue Breathing/ Cardiopulmonary Resuscitation (CPR):** for children 1–8 years old, begin with Step 6, page 35; for children 8+ years old, begin with Step 6, page 41. If the child is breathing, see **When to See a Doctor,** page 112.

Figure 3

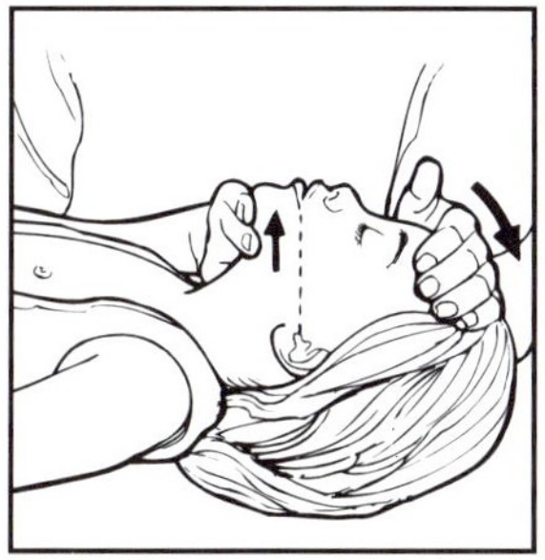

Figure 4

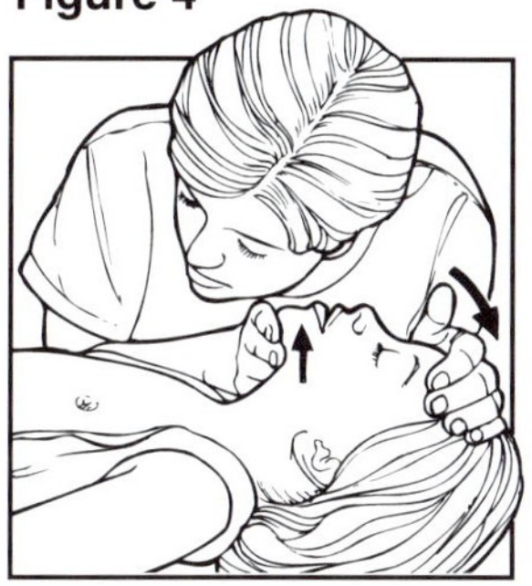

If the Choking Child Is Unconscious (Not Responsive)

1. Check for signs of unconsciousness:

- There is no response when you gently shake the child's shoulder and call her name. (Figure 5)
- The child is limp.
- The child may have a pale, blue, or gray color, and her lips, gums, and nails may be blue.

Figure 5

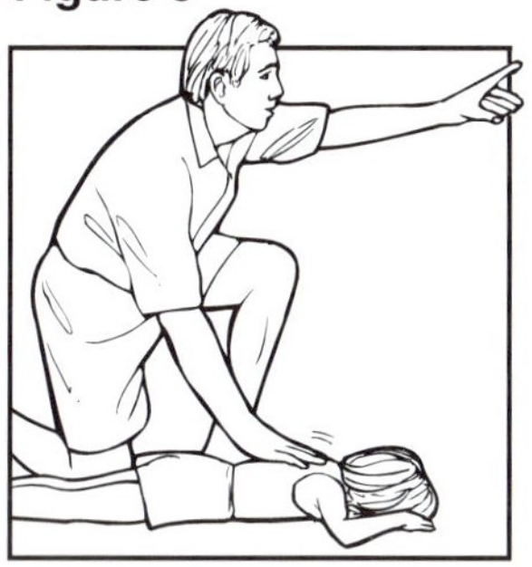

2. Shout for help.

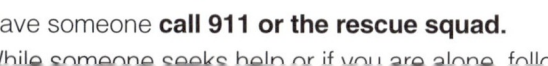

Have someone **call 911 or the rescue squad.**
While someone seeks help or if you are alone, follow

3. Position the child face up.

Support the child's head and neck and turn the child onto her back. (Figure 6)

4. Open the airway.

a. Place one hand on the child's forehead and place the fingers of your other hand on the bony part of the child's chin.

b. Lift the child's chin and tilt her head back. The neck should not be stretched far back. If the child is older than 8 years, tilt her head farther back—her chin should be pointing toward the ceiling. (Figure 7)

5. Check breathing.

While holding the airway open, place your ear over the child's mouth and look at her chest. Look, listen, and feel for breath for 3–5 seconds. (Figure 8)

If the child is not breathing,

proceed to Step 6.

If the child is breathing but not responsive:

a. Position her head to keep the airway open. Use the jaw-thrust technique if there is a possibility of a back or neck injury.

b. If a back or neck injury is not suspected, place the child in the recovery position, as follows:

1. Kneel beside the child.
2. Turn the child onto her side by pulling her toward you.
3. Position the child's head to keep the airway open.

Figure 6

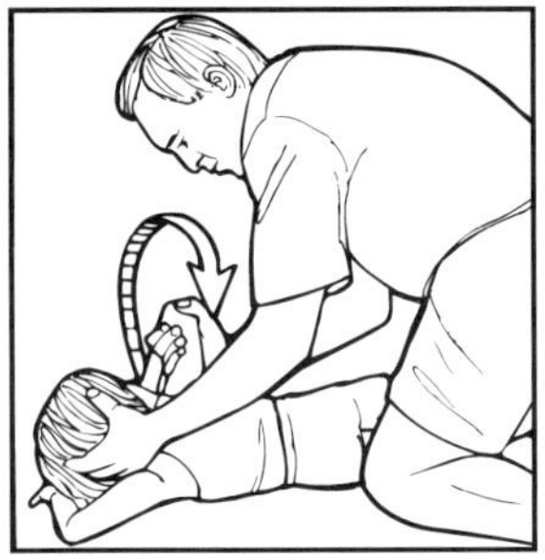

Figure 7

Figure 8

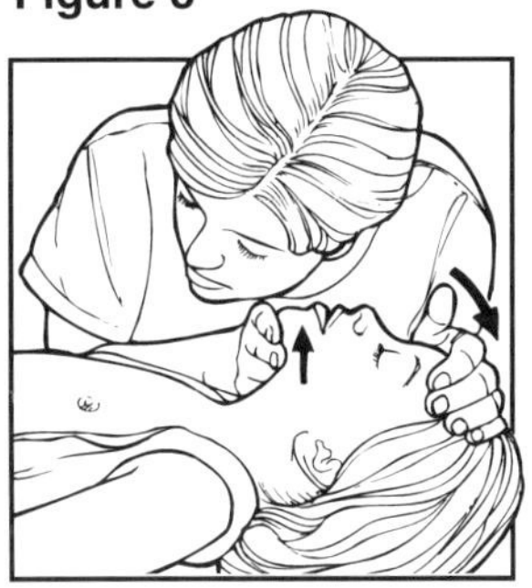

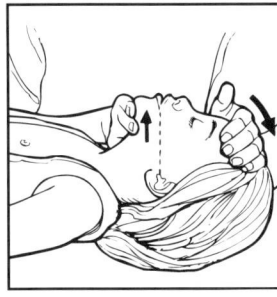

8. Position yourself for abdominal thrusts.

Straddle the child's thighs, without bearing weight on her.

9. Find the correct hand placement for abdominal thrusts.

a. Place the heel of one hand in the middle of the child's abdomen, slightly above the navel (belly-button) and below the rib cage. (Figure 11)

b. Place your other hand on top of the first hand. Raise your fingers up, off the child's abdomen. (If the child is very small, use only one hand to perform abdominal thrusts.)

10. Give five abdominal thrusts.

a. Press inward and upward toward the child's chest. Pause for 1 second between thrusts. Each thrust is an attempt to force out of the windpipe the object that is causing the child to choke. (Figure 12)

b. Adjust the force of the thrusts to the size of the child.

11. Check for the foreign object.

Place your thumb on top of the child's tongue, wrap your fingers under the child's jaw, and pull down the jaw to open the mouth. Look inside the mouth. (Figure 13)

Children 1–8 Years Old

If you see a foreign object: Try to remove it. Use your index finger in a hooked position. Move the finger sideways to sweep the object to the side of the mouth. This will prevent the object from being pushed downward, farther into the throat. (Figure 14)

NOTE: *You may have removed only part of the object. Continue to Step 12 to determine airway clearance.*

Figure 11

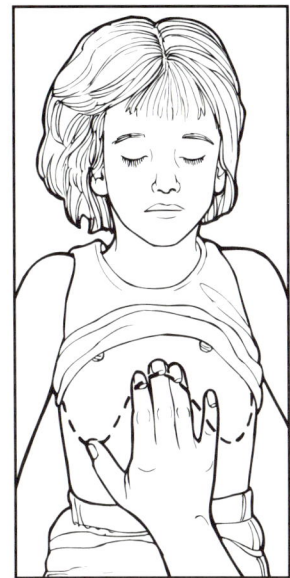

Figure 12

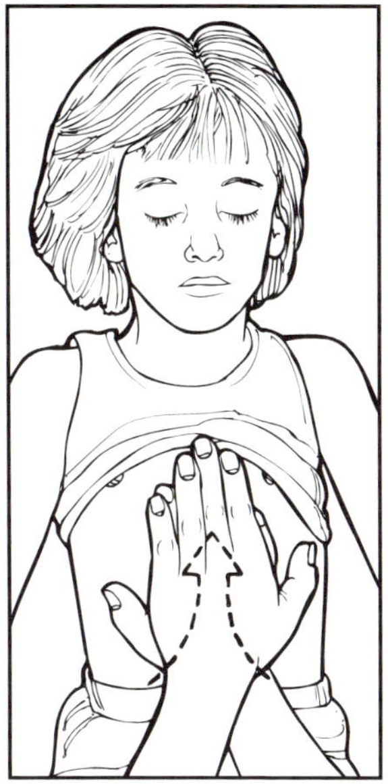

Figure 13

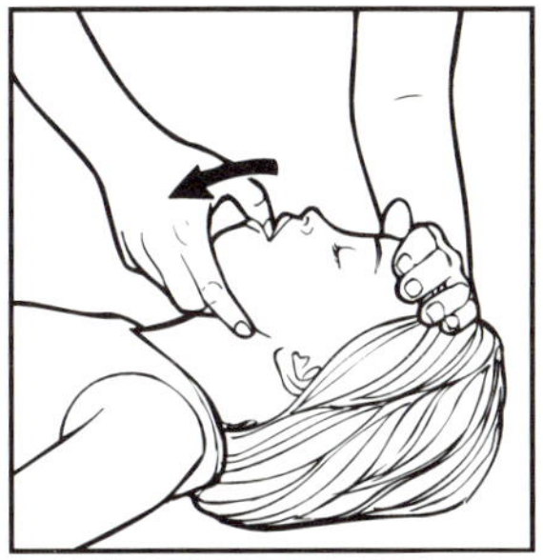

Figure 14

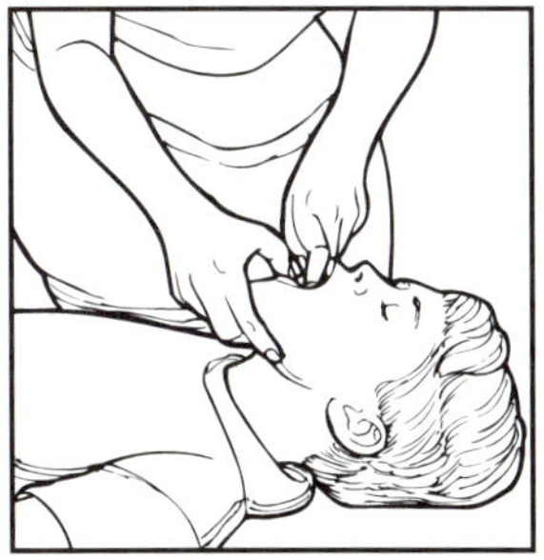

CHOKING: 1+ YEARS

If you do not see an object: Do not probe into the throat as this might push the object farther down into the throat. Proceed to Step 12 instead.

Children 8 Years and Older

Try to remove the foreign object, whether or not you can see it. While holding the child's mouth open, sweep the back of the throat with a hooked finger. (Figure 13). Pull the object out if you can feel it.

NOTE: *You may have removed only part of the object. Continue to Step 12 to determine airway clearance.*

12. Open the airway.

a. Place one hand on the child's forehead and place the fingers of your other hand on the bony part of the child's chin.

b. Lift the child's chin and tilt her head back. The neck should not be stretched far back. If the child is older than 8 years, tilt her head farther back—her chin should be pointing toward the ceiling. (Figure 15)

Figure 15

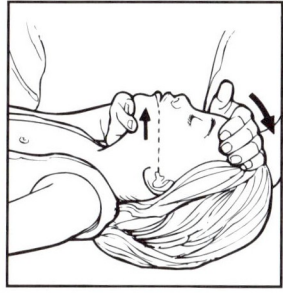

13. Give two rescue breaths.

a. Leaving your hand on the child's forehead, use your thumb and index finger to pinch her nose shut.

b. Place your mouth over the child's mouth, making a tight seal.

c. Give a breath for 1 to $1\frac{1}{2}$ seconds. (Figure 16)

d. Look at or feel the child's chest when giving a breath—the chest should rise.

e. If the breath does not go in easily, reposition the child's head and try again.

f. If the breath still does not go in easily, proceed to Step 14.

Figure 16

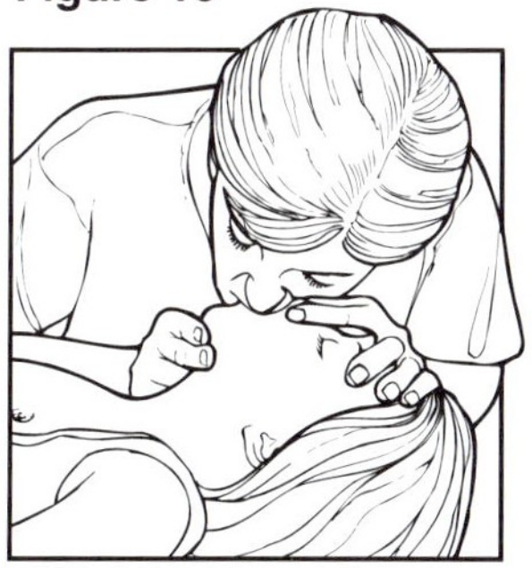

14. Repeat Steps 8–13 three times, as

15. Seek medical assistance.

If three cycles of abdominal thrusts and rescue breaths are unsuccessful, **call 911 or the rescue squad,** if you have not already done so.

16. Repeat Steps 8–13 until:

- the object is dislodged. Proceed to Step 17.
- The child regains consciousness.
- Medical help arrives.

17. Check breathing.

If the child is breathing, see **When to See a Doctor,** page 112.

If the child is not crying or if you are not sure if the child is breathing:

a. Position the child on her back.

b. Open the airway:

1. Place one hand on the child's forehead.
2. Place the fingers of your other hand on the bony part of the chin.
3. Lift the chin and tilt the child's head back. The middle of the back of her head should be flat, and the corner of her mouth should be in line with her earlobe. The neck should not be over-extended or stretched far back.
4. Keep your hand on the child's forehead to keep the airway open.

c. Place your ear over the child's mouth and look at her chest. Look, listen, and feel for a breath for 3–5 seconds. (Figure 17)

Figure 17

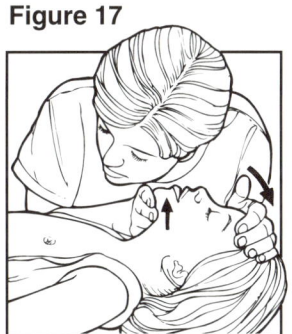

Safety Highlights

Do

- **Do** assume there is a back or neck injury if the child was diving, surfing, sailing, or water skiing.
- **Do** begin rescue breathing as soon as you determine that the child is not breathing.
- **Do** keep the child's neck and body in a straight line as you move the child to shore, onto a dock, and so on.
- **Do** move the child with the assistance of others, if possible.
- **Do** see **Back and Neck Injuries,** page 45, for more information on moving a child.

Don't

- **Don't** bend or twist the child's neck or body.
- **Don't** try to "squeeze" water out of the child's lungs; this is a problem that can be resolved by doctors later.
- **Don't** endanger yourself. Float the child to water shallow enough for you to stand in, or hold onto the side of the pool or boat.

Immediate Action

1. Look at the surroundings and the general appearance of the child.

(Take a few seconds.)

- Is it possible that the child received a severe blow to the head or twisted her back or neck severely (from diving, violently tossing about in a strong wave, or from hitting or being hit by an object)?
- Does the child have an obvious wound on her head?

If the answer to either of these questions is *yes,* the child may have a back or neck injury. Handle the child very carefully. Do not bend or twist her neck or body. Keep her head in line with the rest of her body.

2. Check the child's level of consciousness.

a. Position yourself next to the child in the water.

b. If the child is floating face down, carefully turn the child onto her back, keeping her head in line with her body. Place a hand under the child's back to float her. (Figure 1) If the child is in a tub or a small shallow pool, lift her out and place her on her back on the floor or the ground.

c. Tap the child's shoulder and shout, "Are you okay?"

If there is no response and the child appears to be unconscious,

proceed to Step 3 without bending or twisting the child's neck or body.

If the child is responsive and you do not suspect a back or neck injury,

remove the child from the water and sit the child in an upright position. If the child has to vomit, assist her. Keep the child quiet and warm by wrapping her in a towel or blanket. See **When to See a Doctor,** page 118.

If the child is responsive and you suspect a back or neck injury,

remain in the water with the child and have someone **call 911 or the rescue squad.** While awaiting medical assistance, prevent the child from moving. If the child vomits, carefully support her head, keeping it in line with her body, and turn the child onto her side. Clear the child's mouth. Support the child on her back until medical assistance arrives.

Figure 1

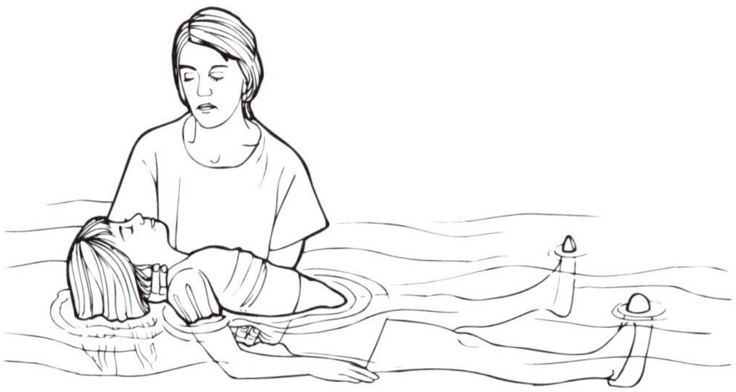

3. Seek medical assistance.

Have someone **call 911 or the rescue squad.** While someone seeks help or if you are alone, stay with the child and proceed with the following steps.

4. Open the airway.

a. Place one hand on the child's forehead and place your other hand on the bony part of the child's chin.

b. Lift the child's chin gently while pressing down on the forehead to carefully tilt the head back. If you are still in the water and it will take some time before you are able to transport the child to a flat surface, perform this step in the water. (Figure 2)

NOTE: *If a back or neck injury is suspected, do not move the child's head. Place two or three fingers under each side of the child's lower jaw and lift upward (jaw-thrust technique). (Figure 3)*

5. Check breathing.

Look at the child's chest and feel and listen for air movement from her mouth or nose. Check for 3–5 seconds. (Figure 4)

If the child is breathing but not responsive,

maintain an open airway and proceed to Step 7.

If the child is not breathing:

a. Maintain an open airway by keeping one hand on the child's forehead and your other hand under the child's back, supporting the child if she is in the water.

b. Give two rescue breaths.

1. For an infant, 0–1 year, cover the infant's mouth and nose tightly with your mouth. For a child 1+ years, use the thumb and index finger of the hand that is on the child's forehead to pinch the

Figure 2

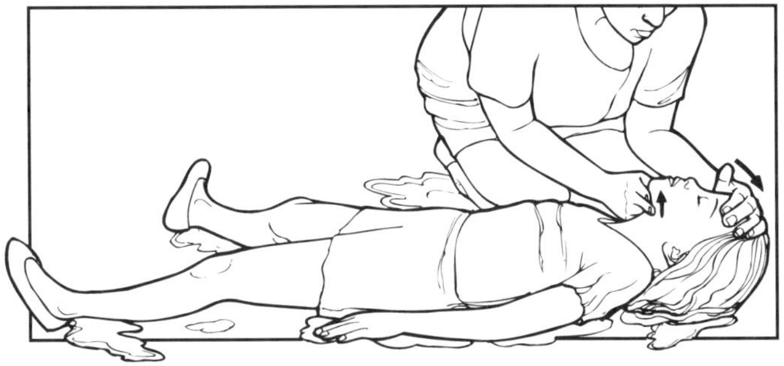

Figure 3

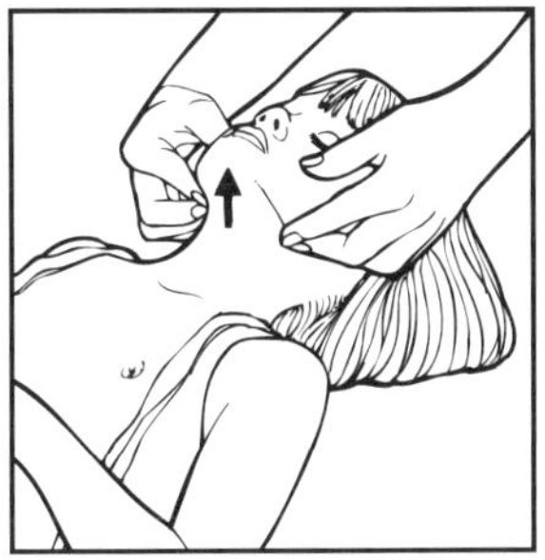

Figure 4

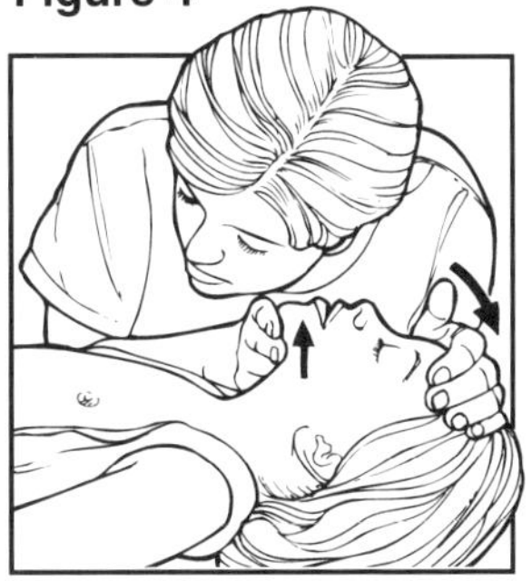

b. Once out of the water, position the child on her back, maintaining an open airway and continuing rescue breathing. (Figure 9) If you are alone, perform rescue breathing for 1 minute, then **call 911 or the rescue squad** if you have not already done so.

c. Recheck breathing.

d. Continue rescue breaths until breathing resumes or until medical help arrives.

If no pulse is present,

a. Without bending or twisting the child's neck or body, carefully move the child to a flat surface.

b. Begin cardiopulmonary resuscitation (CPR). (Figure 10) Do not tilt the child's head back. See **Rescue Breathing/Cardiopulmonary Resuscitation (CPR):** 0–1 year, page 27; 1–8 years, page 33; 8+ years, page 39.

c. Perform CPR for 1 minute, then **call 911 or the rescue squad** if you have not already done so.

d. Recheck breathing and pulse.

e. Continue CPR, or rescue breathing, until breathing and pulse are restored or until medical help arrives.

7. Keep the airway clear.

a. If the child vomits at any point, carefully support her head, keeping it in line with her body, and turn the child onto her side. (Figure 11)

b. Clear the child's mouth.

c. Roll the child onto her back.

d. Recheck breathing and pulse.

e. Resume rescue breathing or CPR as necessary.

8. If breathing and pulse are present, treat for shock.

See **Shock,** page 169.

Figure 9

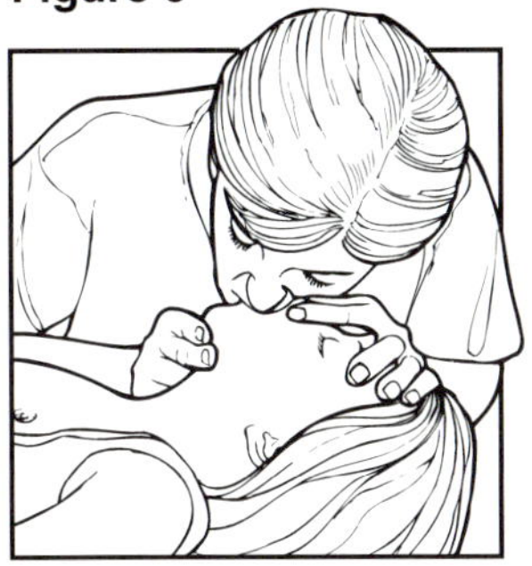

Figure 10

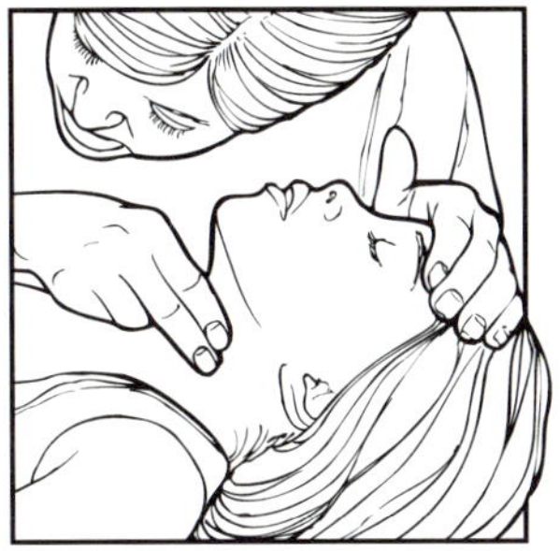

Figure 11

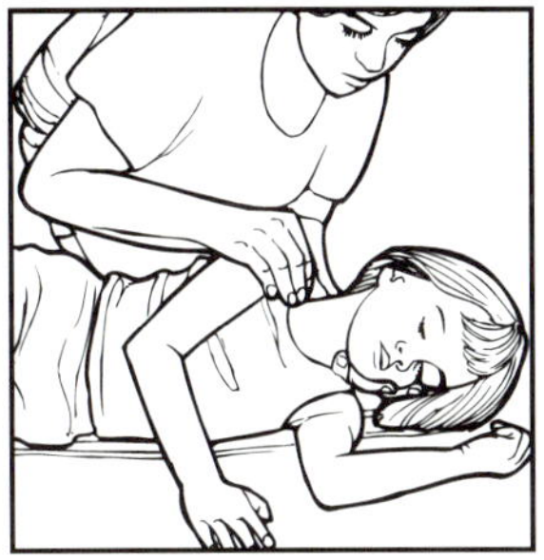

When to See a Doctor

Call 911 or the rescue squad if previously instructed to do so. Otherwise, take the child to see a doctor immediately, especially if either of the following applies:

- The child was in very cold water, even for a short time, before being rescued—he may have hypothermia. Symptoms include continuous or violent shivering, slow or slurred speech, confusion, difficulty walking, and lack of coordination. Symptoms may progress to muscle spasms, body rigidity, and unconsciousness.
- The child revives but had lost consciousness, breathing ability, or pulse.

Home Treatment

If the child did not lose consciousness during the incident, keep the child warm with blankets or towels and observe her for breathing difficulty or symptoms of hypothermia (violent shivering, slow or slurred speech, confusion, difficulty walking, and lack of coordination). If the child develops symptoms of a cold or chest congestion within the following week, call the doctor. The child should be evaluated to determine if water inhaled into the lungs caused an infection or other problems.

Safety Highlights

Do

- **Do** request help from others while you transport the child—the child may be angry and combative.
- **Do** provide emotional support to the child.
- **Do** continuously observe the child for breathing difficulty.
- **Do** protect the child from harming himself or herself.

Don't

- **Don't** cause the child to panic.
- **Don't** scold or ridicule the child, because it may lead to depression.
- **Don't** leave the child alone.

Immediate Action

1. Look at the surroundings and the general appearance of the child.

(Take a few seconds.)

- Is there evidence of drugs near the child (pills, powder, syringe, liquor container, and so on)? (Figure 1)
- Is there evidence of a substance in the child's mouth or nose, or needle marks on her skin?
- Did a witness report seeing the child take a drug?

If the answer to any of the above signs is *yes,* the child may have overdosed on a drug or a combination of drugs and alcohol.

Figure 1

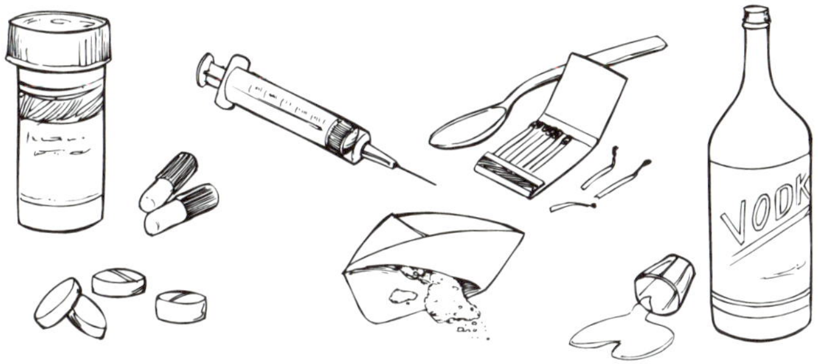

4. If a drug overdose is suspected, call the Poison Control Center.

Phone # ______________________________

If there is no Poison Control Center in your area, call the child's doctor,

Phone # ______________________________

OR

the local hospital emergency department.

Phone # ______________________________

If available, bring evidence of the drug that caused the overdose to the phone.

a. Describe the child's symptoms and the evidence of drugs you have found.

b. Write down and follow the instructions you are given.

5. Stimulate vomiting if you are instructed to do so.

If the child is awake and alert, and if the Poison Control Center, doctor, or hospital emergency personnel instruct you to do so, stimulate vomiting.

a. Give the child syrup of ipecac (available at most drugstores). (Figure 4)

b. Follow syrup of ipecac with one or two glasses of warm water.

c. Have the child vomit into a bucket or bowl so you can retain a sample for medical evaluation.

d. If there is no vomiting within 30 minutes, repeat Steps a and b.

e. If there is no vomiting within the *next* 30 minutes, do not repeat. Tickle the back of the child's throat with your finger to stimulate vomiting. Remember to have the child vomit into a bucket or bowl so you can retain a sample.

Syrup of Ipecac Dosage Chart

0–1 year	2 teaspoons
1–8 years	1 tablespoon
9+ years	2 tablespoons

Figure 4

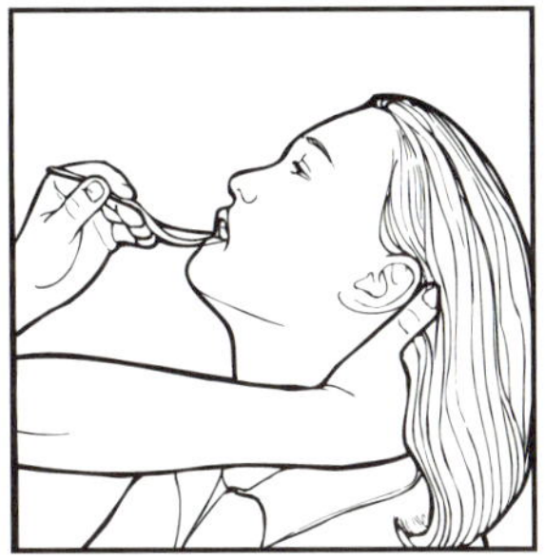

6. Keep the child awake.

Stay with the child; keep her awake and moving by involving her in an activity or talking. It may be helpful to play music. Avoid the use of caffeine or other stimulants as they may make the child's drug reaction worse.

7. Provide emotional support to the child.

Reassure the child. (Figure 5) Do not scold or ridicule her, as this may lead to depression. Do not panic the child—she may become violent.

Figure 5

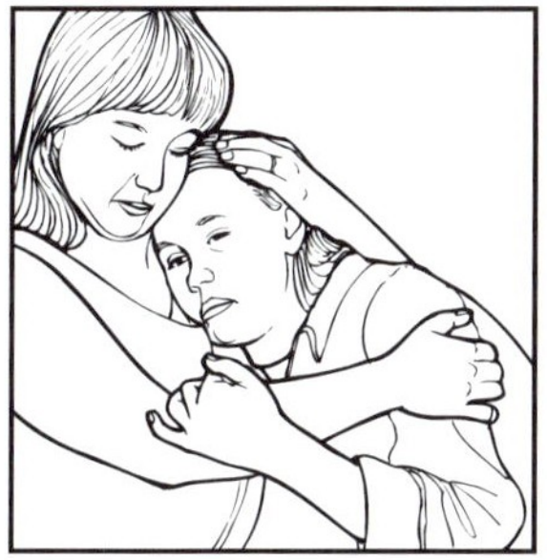

8. Transport the child to a medical facility if:

- You are instructed to do so by the Poison Control Center, the child's doctor, or the hospital emergency department.
- The child is becoming increasingly drowsy.
- The child behaves violently or is panicky.
- The child becomes severely depressed.

9. Call 911 or the rescue squad if the child becomes unconscious.

See **Rescue Breathing/Cardiopulmonary Resuscitation (CPR):** 0–1 year, page 27; 1–8 years, page 33; 8+ years, page 39.

When to See a Doctor

Take the child to see a doctor if any of the following apply:

- You are instructed to do so by the Poison Control Center, the child's doctor, or the hospital emergency department.
- There is not a Poison Control Center in your area, the child's doctor is not available by phone, and you know or suspect that the child has suffered a drug overdose.
- The child is becoming increasingly drowsy.
- The child behaves violently or is panicky.
- The child becomes severely depressed.

Regardless of symptoms, the child should eventually see a doctor, especially if a drug dependency problem might exist.

Home Treatment

1. Treat the child as directed by the Poison Control Center, the doctor, or the hospital emergency department.
2. Seek drug and/or psychotherapeutic counseling for the child to provide appropriate professional attention to the emotional and physical issues related to drug dependency and/or abuse.

Safety Highlights

Do

- **Do** report all signs of illness when reporting a fever to the child's doctor.
- **Do** keep the child in a cool environment, but avoid drafts.
- **Do** encourage rest and quiet activity.

Don't

- **Don't** bundle the child in extra clothes and blankets, even if the child has the chills.
- **Don't** give aspirin to a child who may have the flu, chicken pox, or an unknown illness.
- **Don't** try to reduce a fever by sponging the child with alcohol.

Immediate Action

Doctors differ in how and at what point they want a fever controlled. If your doctor has advised you to reduce the child's fever by giving acetaminophen and/or "sponging" the child, do the following:

1. Check the child's temperature.

Use an oral, rectal, digital, or ear thermometer to measure the child's temperature. See **Checking Temperature,** page 16, for method and to determine which thermometer to use.

Range of Normal Temperatures	
Oral	97.6°–98.6°F
Axillary	97°–98°F
Rectal	99°–99.6°F

Note: Everyone's body temperature is higher with activity, is lowest in the morning, and is highest in the late afternoon.

2. Give the child acetaminophen according to the doctor's instructions.

Acetaminophen dosage depends on the weight of the child. For an infant, you can put the medication into a nipple and let her suck it. It is wise to have acetaminophen rectal suppositories available in addition to the oral forms. If the child repeatedly vomits, is very drowsy, or unconscious, the rectal suppository should be given; follow the dosage instructions on the label or ask the pharmacist how much of the suppository to give. Apply a lubricant such as petroleum jelly to the suppository and gently insert it into child's rectum.

NOTE: *Aspirin should not be given to children with chicken pox or flu. It is best avoided if you do not know the cause of the child's illness.*

Acetaminophen Dosage Chart

Age	Weight (in pounds)	80 milligram drops, 0.8 milliliters per dropperful (dppr.)	160 milligram elixir, 5 milliliters per teaspoon	80 milligram chewable tablets	160 milligram junior-strength tablets
0–3 mo.	6–11 lb.	½ dppr. (0.4 ml)	—	—	—
4–11 mo.	12–17 lb.	1 dppr. (0.8 ml)	½ teaspoon	1 tablet	—
12–23 mo.	18–23 lb.	1½ dppr. (1.2 ml)	¾ teaspoon	1½ tablets	—
2–3 yr.	24–35 lb.	2 dppr. (1.6 ml)	1 teaspoon	2 tablets	—
4–5 yr.	36–47 lb.	—	1½ teaspoons	3 tablets	—
6–8 yr.	48–59 lb.	—	2 teaspoons	4 tablets	2 tablets
9–10 yr.	60–71 lb.	—	2½ teaspoons	5 tablets	2½ tablets
11 yr.	72–95 lb.	—	3 teaspoons	6 tablets	3 tablets
12–14 yr.	96 lb. and over	—	—	—	4 tablets

3. Sponge bathe the child to reduce fever.

Place the child in a tub of shallow, lukewarm water. Most of her body should be exposed to the air. Sponge the child for 15–20 minutes. Sponge her head and underarms to bring the fever down more quickly. (Figure 1)

Figure 1

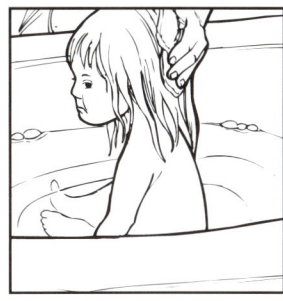

4. Dry the child and dress her lightly.

5. Give the child liquids if she is awake and alert.

Fever can easily result in dehydration. Therefore, frequent administration of liquids—including water, juices, gelatin, ices, and so on—is recommended.

When to See a Doctor

Doctors differ in how and at what point they want a fever controlled. Ask the child's doctor about his or her recommendations. Some general guidelines with which most pediatricians agree are as follows.

Call the child's doctor if:

- The child is under 4 months and either rectal or axillary temperature is over 100°F.
- The child is between 4 months and 2 years and either rectal or axillary temperature is over 102°F.
- The child has a fever between 105° and 106°F that cannot be brought down by acetaminophen.
- The child has a fever of 106°F or over.
- The child has any temperature 1–2 degrees above normal for 24 hours.

Safety Highlights

Do

- **Do** assess the injury before moving the child.
- **Do** assess the child's level of consciousness, breathing ability, and pulse if the child was in a serious accident; other parts of the body also may have been injured.
- **Do** question the child about how the injury occurred.
- **Do** act in a calm manner to keep the child still and calm and to help the child's muscles relax.

Don't

- **Don't** move the child if you suspect a back or neck injury.
- **Don't** move an injured extremity; keep it in the same position in which you found it.
- **Don't** try to straighten an injured limb.
- **Don't** try to push a broken bone back under the skin.
- **Don't** put pressure on top of a wound.
- **Don't** let the child move the injured part.

Immediate Action

1. Look at the surroundings and general appearance of the child.

(Take a few seconds.)

- Was there a severe fall (perhaps from a tree, from playground equipment, or out of a window)?
- Was the child thrown from a motor vehicle or bicycle?
- Was there a forceful blow to the injured area, or was the area twisted?
- Was the child physically handled in a rough, forceful manner?
- Is a bone sticking out of the child's skin? (Figure 1)

Figure 1

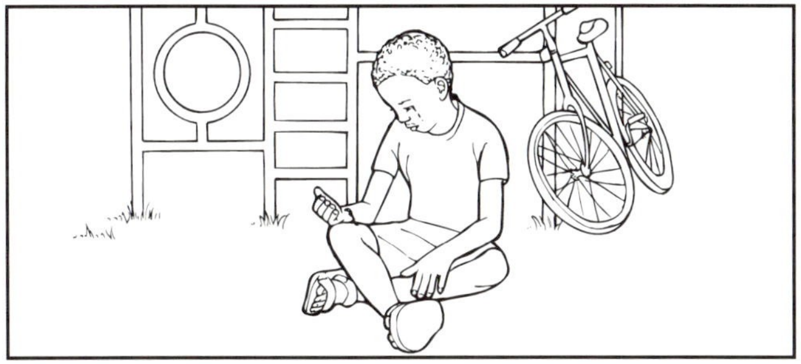

If the answer to any of the above is *yes,* the child could have a fracture (broken bone). Handle the child very carefully, without moving the injured part.

2. Check for and treat the most life-threatening problems now.

Check for signs of unconsciousness, no breathing, no pulse, bleeding, and shock. (Figure 2) See **Life-Threat Checklist,** page 23.

Call 911 or the rescue squad as recommended in **Life-Threat Checklist,** page 23.

NOTE: *If there is profuse bleeding and you suspect a broken bone, press on the nearest pressure point located between the heart and the wound.* *See **If Bleeding Cannot Be Immediately Controlled,** pages 66–69.*

Once the most life-threatening problems have been attended to, you may proceed with further treatment as instructed below.

Figure 2

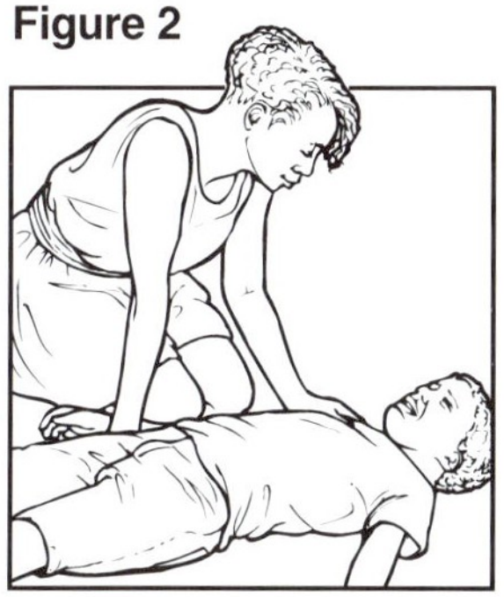

3. Check for signs of a fracture.

a. Look at the injured area carefully.

b. Touch the area gently to check for pain, and ask the child to point to the most painful area. (Figure 3)

c. Suspect a fracture if any of the following applies:

- An extremity (arm, leg, finger, toe) is blue or pale.
- The nail beds are blue or pale.
- An extremity is swollen.
- An extremity is bruised.
- An extremity is crooked or deformed.
- An extremity is cold.
- An extremity is numb.
- An extremity is painful.
- An extremity is unable to bear weight or is not usable.

Figure 3

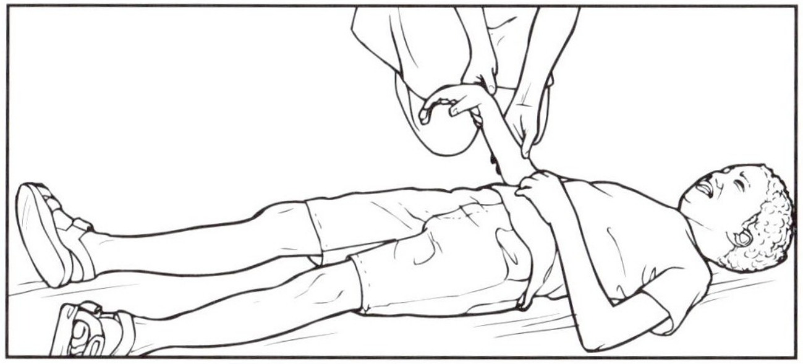

- A "snap" was heard at the time of injury.
- A bone is sticking out of the skin.
- There is pain in the groin, lower abdomen, or hip area, which may be from a fractured pelvis.

See **Back and Neck Injuries,** page 45, for signs of and care for an injured back or neck.

NOTE: *The child may have all or only some of the signs listed above. A sprain results from the twisting, stretching, or tearing of ligaments around a joint and has many of the same symptoms as a fracture, which is a broken bone. An X ray is usually required to determine whether the injury is a sprain or a fracture. It is therefore safest to treat the injury as if it were a fracture and have the child see a doctor, who may order an X ray.*

4. Protect the wound, if any.

a. Do not touch any bone that is sticking out of the skin.

b. Gently cover the bone and wound with sterile gauze or a clean cloth. (Figure 4) Secure the gauze or cloth gently with tape or strips of cloth. You should be able to slide a finger beneath the gauze or cloth.

Figure 4

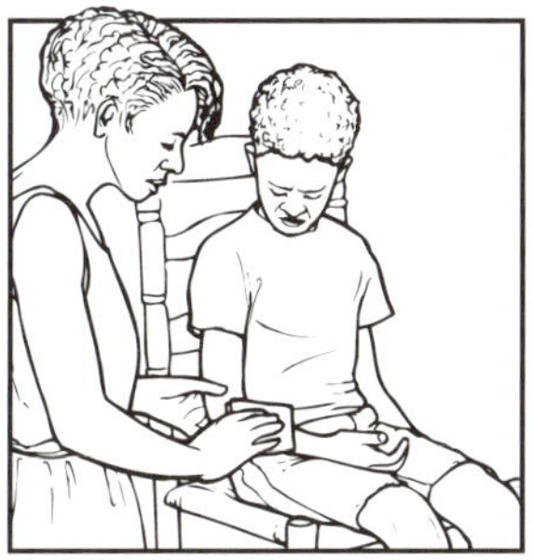

5. Immobilize the injured part.

(Hold it still.)

a. Do not try to straighten the injured limb; keep it in the same position in which it was found.

b. Carry out the steps for immobilizing specific bones and joints as given in **Splinting Techniques,** pages 134–140. (Figure 5)

Figure 5

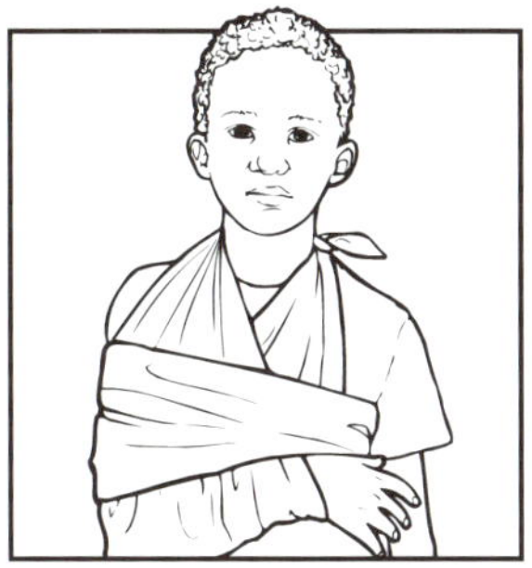

6. Seek medical assistance.

a. **Call 911 or the rescue squad** if the child may have a fracture of the pelvis, hip, or upper leg, or a back or neck injury.

Application of a Splint

1. Pad the splint with cloth.
2. Secure the padded splint to the extremity with strips of cloth, scarves, ties, belts, or whatever else is available. Place the strips above and below the break, but not *on* the break. Tie knots in the strips on the side of the injured extremity, not on the top or bottom.
3. Tie the splint firmly, but you should be able to feel a pulse in the injured area. Loosen the splint if the extremity becomes cold, numb, or blue or pale.

Slings

A *sling* holds an injured arm up against the chest, in a bent position, preventing shoulder and elbow movement.

Items to Use for Slings

Scarf, tie, shirt, towel, cloth, or other triangular bandage (Safety pins are helpful in securing the sling.)

Application of a Sling

1. Position the child's arm across his chest in a bent, diagonal position, with the fingers resting higher on the chest than the elbow.
2. Slide one end of the sling under the affected arm and pull the corner of the sling up along the side of the child's neck, directly above his fingers. (Figure 7)
3. Bring the other end of the sling over the arm, and pull the corner of the sling up toward the back and to the side of the child's neck, enclosing the arm. (Figure 8)
4. Tie a knot with the two ends of the sling. (Figure 9)

Figure 7

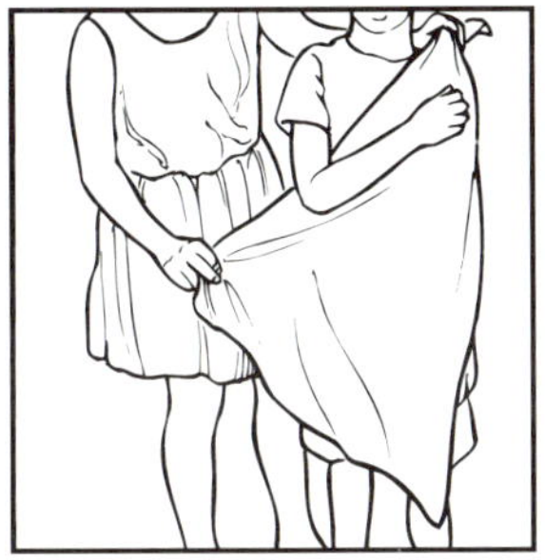

Figure 8

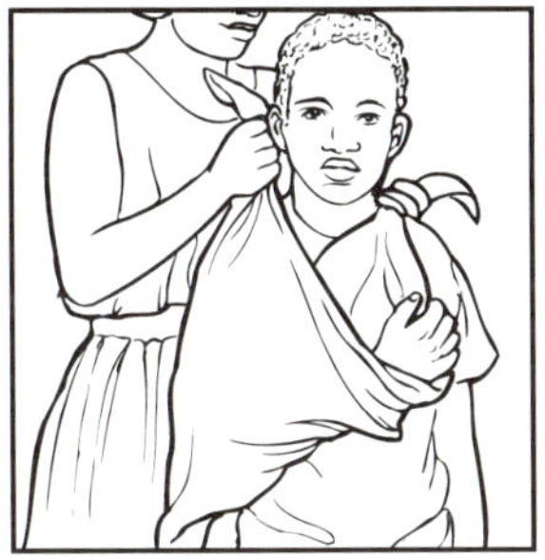

Figure 9

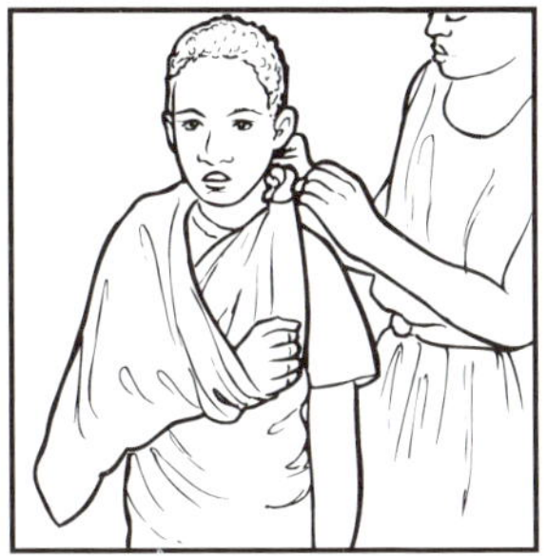

5. Adjust the sling as necessary.
   - The sling should support the weight of the arm, with the fingers resting higher on the chest than the elbow.
   - To prevent the elbow from slipping out of the sling you may tie a knot or use a safety pin to secure the lower outside corner of the cloth. (Figure 10)
   - Leave the fingers exposed so that they can be examined for adequate circulation.
   - For additional support, secure the sling by tying a wide cloth over the sling and around the child's body. (Figure 11)

Figure 10

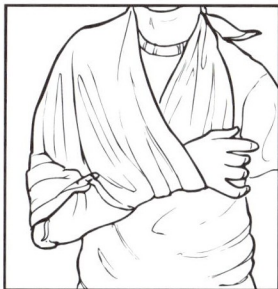

Figure 11

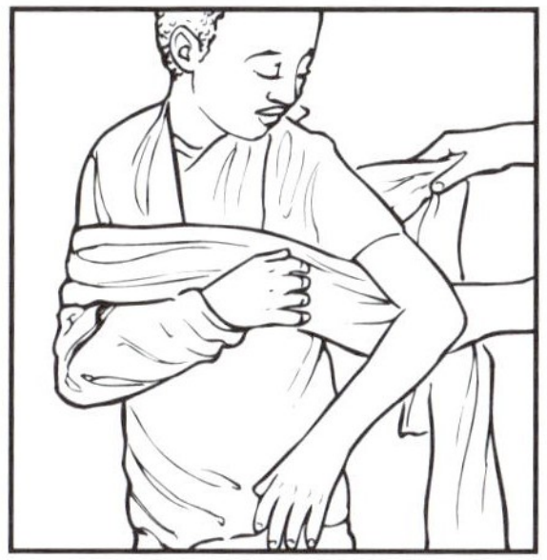

Splinting Techniques

Collarbone and Shoulder

1. Apply a sling to the arm associated with the injured collarbone or shoulder for support. Position the sling so the child's hand rests 4–5 inches higher than his elbow. (Figure 10)
2. Tie a wide cloth around the child's body, over the sling, to hold the arm against the body. (Figure 11)

Upper Arm

1. Place a pad (such as a small folded towel) under the child's injured arm. The arm should be held against the side of the body, with the lower arm across the chest.
2. Place a padded splint along the outer side of the child's upper arm.
3. Wrap the splint snugly with strips of cloth. (Figure 12)

Figure 12

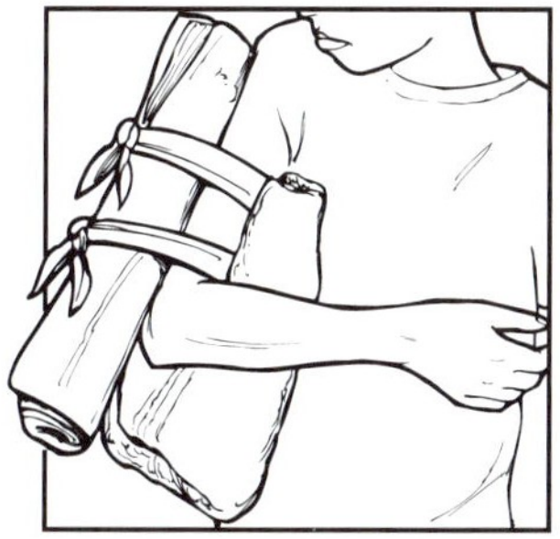

4. Apply a sling for support of the child's lower arm. If a triangular bandage or large cloth is used, use a safety pin to hold the loose ends together or tie a knot. (Figure 13)
5. Tie a wide cloth around the child's body, over the sling, to hold the arm against the body. (Figure 11, above)

Lower Arm, Wrist, or Hand

1. Place a padded splint along the underside of the child's lower arm, or enclose the lower arm in a magazine.
2. Wrap the splint or magazine snugly with cloth. (Figure 14)
3. Apply a sling for support. Position the sling so the child's hand rests 4–5 inches higher than his elbow. (Figure 15)
4. If the arm may be broken, tie a wide cloth around the child's body, over the sling, to hold the arm against the body. (Figure 16)

Bent Elbow

1. Place a padded splint along the underside of the bent elbow.
2. Wrap the splint snugly with cloth, interlacing the cloth in a figure-eight pattern. (Figure 17)
3. Apply a sling for support. Position the sling so the child's hand rests 4–5 inches higher than his elbow. (Figure 18)
4. Tie a cloth around the child's body, over the sling, to hold the arm against the body.

Figure 13

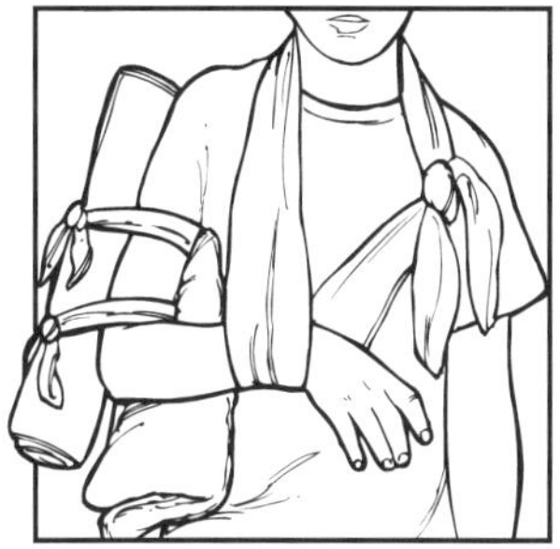

Figure 14

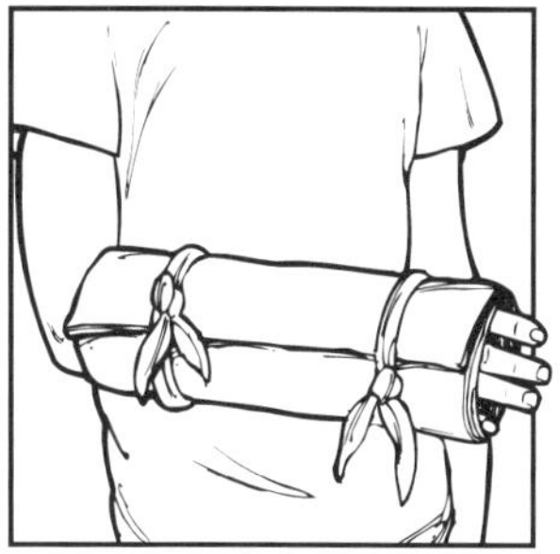

Figure 15

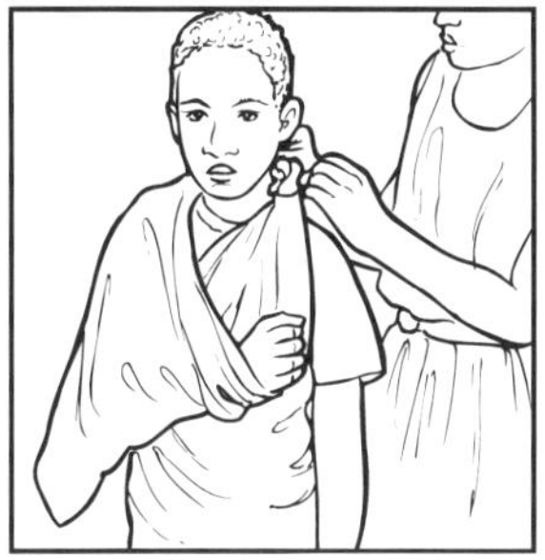

Figure 16

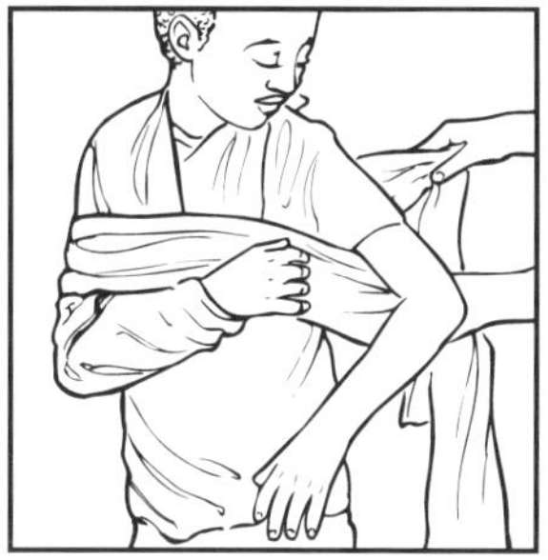

Figure 17

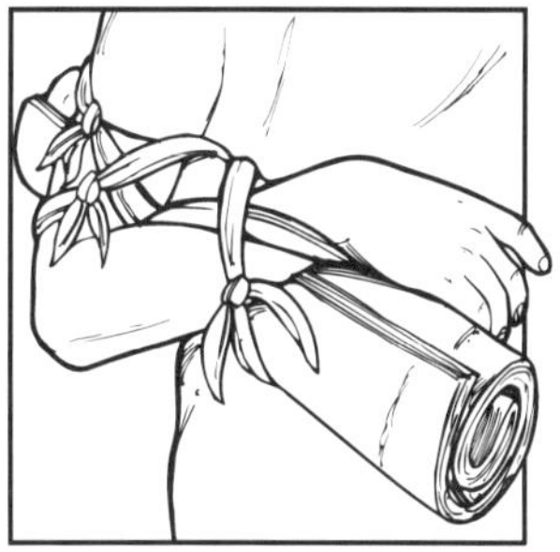

Figure 18

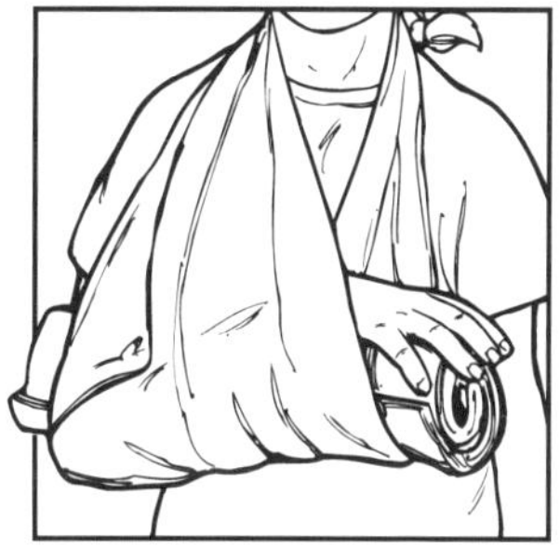

If medical help is not available and you must move the child yourself, do the following:

- Apply long padded splints. Place one splint on the outside of the child's body, from the armpit to below the heel. Place the other splint along the inside of the leg from the crotch to below the heel. Wrap the splints snugly with cloths. The knots should be on the splint, not on top of the leg. (Figure 23)

OR

- Splint the legs together. Place thick padding between the child's legs, along the entire length of the legs. Tie the legs together with strips of cloth. Do this firmly enough to prevent movement. (Figure 24)

If the injured leg is bent, follow the instructions for a fractured pelvis. See **Pelvis,** below.

Pelvis

1. Check for a fracture by gently touching the child in the hip areas, noting where the child feels pain. (Figure 25)
2. **Call 911 or the rescue squad** for transport to a medical facility.
3. Do not allow the child to move her legs.
   a. Leave the legs in the position found—bent or straight.
   b. Place thick padding between the thighs.
   c. Wrap strips of cloth around the legs at the knees and ankles to keep the legs together. (Figure 26)
4. While awaiting medical assistance, treat for shock. See **Shock,** page 169.

Figure 23

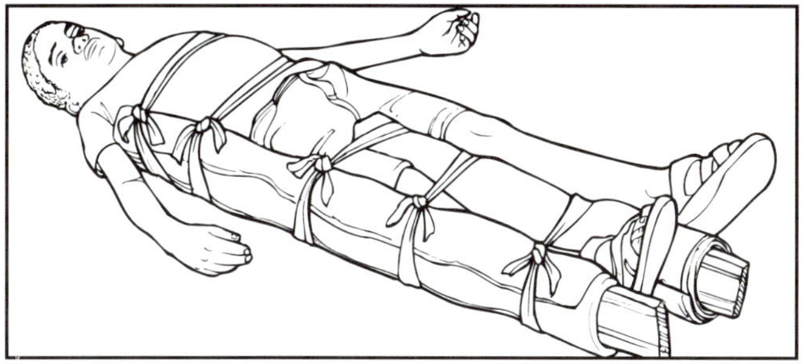

Figure 24

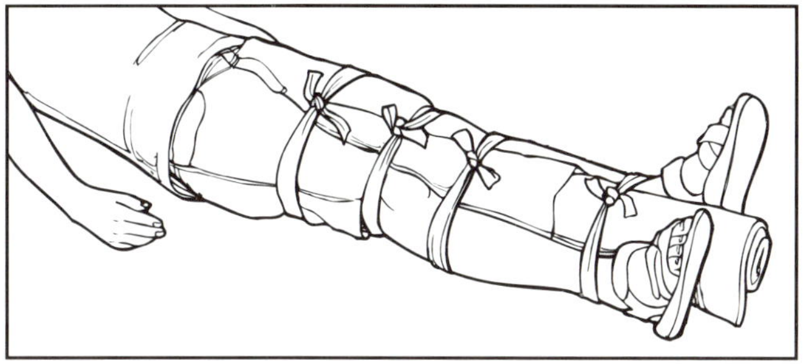

Figure 25

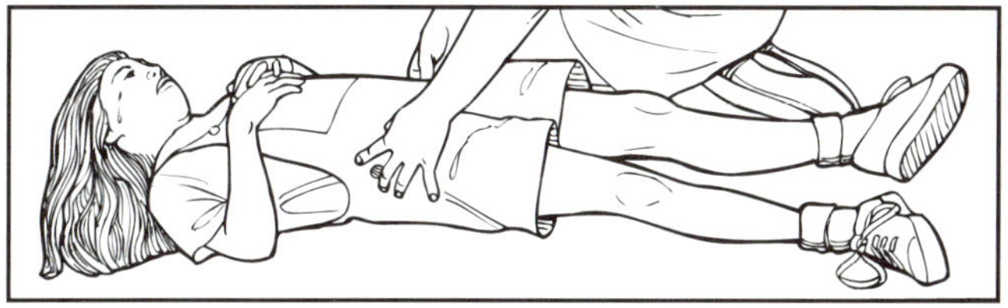

Figure 26

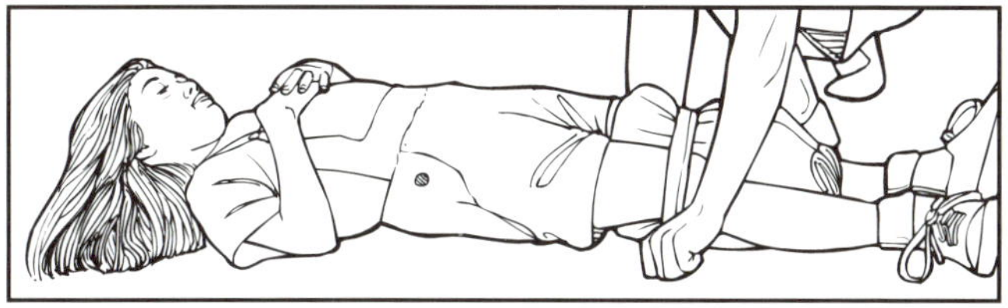

If medical help is not available and you must move the child yourself, do the following:

1. Splint the pelvis as described in Step 3, above.
2. Obtain assistance from other people.
3. Keeping the child's pelvis and legs firmly aligned, carefully roll the child as a unit (all body parts in line) onto her side. (Figure 27)
4. Place a firm object, large enough for the child to lie on, along the child's back (a door, board, ironing board, and so on). If a firm object is unavailable, a blanket may be used.
5. Carefully roll the child, as a unit, onto the object. (Figure 28)
6. Secure the child to the object with strips of cloth, belts, or whatever else is available.
7. Transport the child to the closest medical facility. If using a blanket, have several assistants hold the blanket taut and carry the child to safety; do not drag the child when using a blanket.

Bent Knee

1. Place two padded splints on opposite sides of the child's bent knee.
2. Wrap the splints snugly with strips of cloth. Do not place cloths directly over the broken area; instead, secure the cloths above and below the fracture. (Figure 29)
3. Apply ice, wrapped in plastic or cloth, to the knee.

OR

1. Have the child bend her other knee, at the same angle as the injured knee.
2. Place thick padding between the child's legs, at the thighs and the calves.

Figure 27

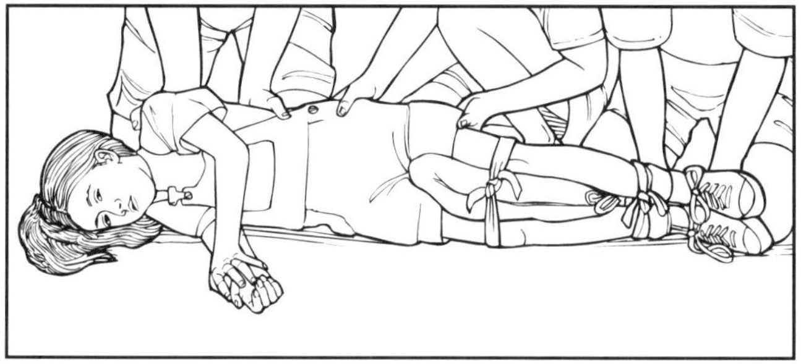

Figure 28

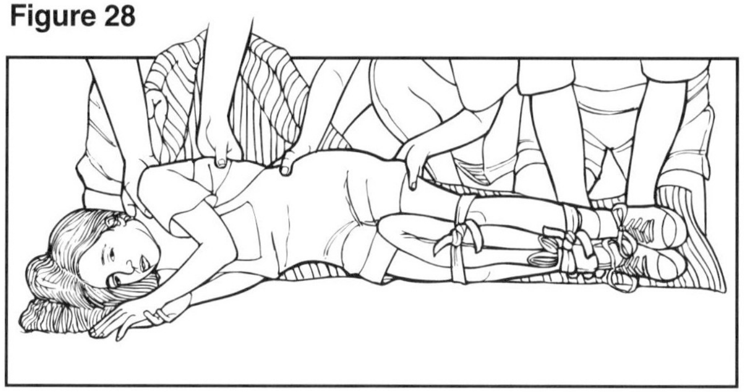

Figure 29

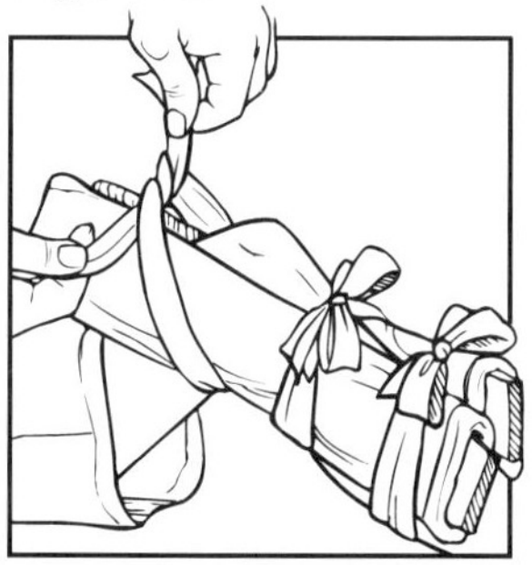

3. Tie the child's legs together with strips of cloth, at the middle of the thighs and the middle of the calves. (Figure 30)
4. Apply ice, wrapped in plastic or cloth, to the knee.

Straight Knee

1. Place a padded splint along the underside of the child's leg, from the top of the thigh to below the heel. Place extra padding under the knee.
2. Wrap the splint snugly with strips of cloth. Do not place cloths directly over the broken area; instead, secure the cloths above and below the fracture. (Figure 31)
3. Apply ice, wrapped in plastic or cloth, to the knee.

Lower Leg

1. Place a padded splint under the child's leg, from the top of the thigh to below the heel.
2. Wrap the splint snugly with strips of cloth, securing the knots on the outside edge of the splint. Do not place cloths directly over the broken area; instead, secure the cloths above and below the fracture. (Figure 31)
3. Apply ice, wrapped in plastic or in cloth, to the injured leg.

OR

1. Place thick padding between the child's legs, along the entire length of the legs.
2. Tie the legs together with strips of cloth. The knots should be between the two legs or on the uninjured leg. (Figure 32)
3. Apply ice, wrapped in plastic or cloth, to the injured leg.

Figure 30

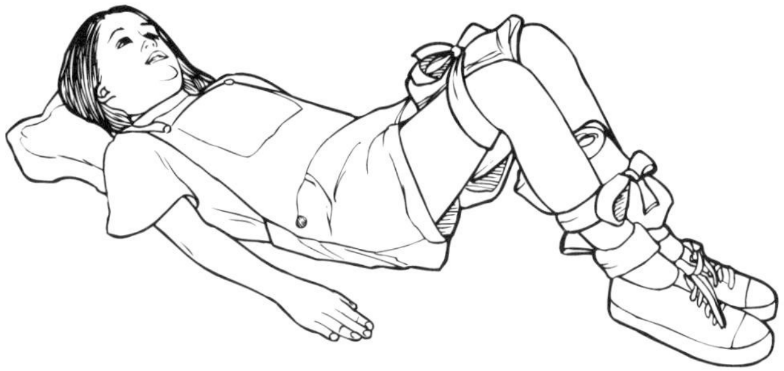

Figure 31

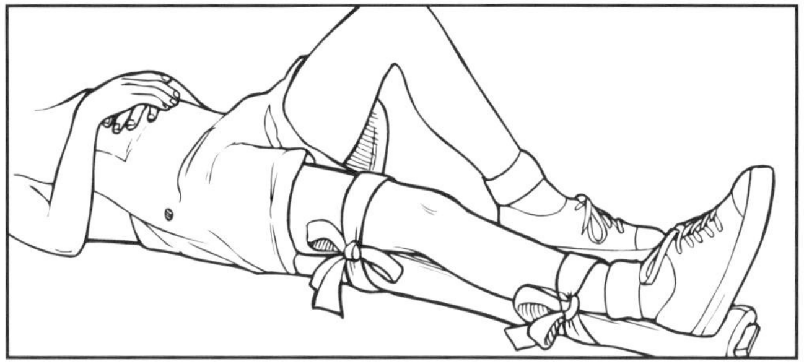

Figure 32

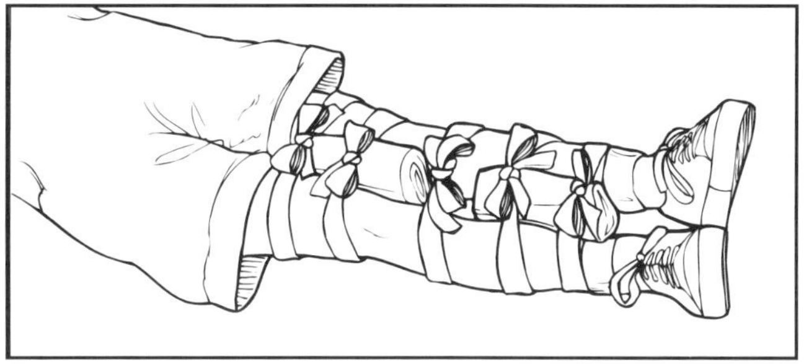

Home Treatment

If the child has marked swelling, bruising, and pain at the site of injury, but has none of the other symptoms noted above, he or she may have a sprain. This occurs when a ligament, which is a tissue that holds bones together, is twisted, stretched, or torn. Mild sprains can be treated at home. However, a "hairline" (small) fracture may be present but not immediately evident. As with all fractures, a hairline fracture should not be treated at home. Therefore, symptoms should be observed carefully over a 48-hour period and the child should be brought to see a doctor if a hairline fracture is suspected.

Home treatment for a sprain is as follows:

1. Apply ice wrapped in a towel to the injured area for at least 30 minutes after the injury occurs. If swelling remains, continue applying ice—on for 30 minutes, off for 15 minutes, on for 30 minutes, and so on, for a few hours.
2. Splint, elevate, and rest the injured extremity for at least 48 hours.
3. The child's parent or guardian should medicate for pain with acetaminophen according to the dosage instructions on the label.
4. If pain and inability to use the limb continue for more than 48 hours, call the child's doctor for further instructions.
5. Allow 4–6 weeks for complete healing of a sprain. Elastic bandages may help relieve symptoms, but do not provide support. Therefore, they are most effective when used in conjunction with a supportive device, such as a splint. Do not apply such bandages so tightly that the area beneath the bandage becomes cold, blue or pale, or numb.

Safety Highlights

Do

- **Do** press lightly when controlling bleeding from a head wound.
- **Do** note how long the child remains unconscious.
- **Do** check the child for injuries to other parts of the body.
- **Do** place the child on his or her side if he or she is vomiting. If the child is unconscious, see **Back and Neck Injuries: If the Child Is Vomiting or Is Bleeding From the Mouth,** page 50, for proper moving techniques.

Don't

- **Don't** move the child if he or she is unconscious, unless he or she is vomiting, is not breathing or has no pulse, and is lying face down. See **Back and Neck Injuries: If the Child Is Lying Face Down and Is Not Breathing or Has No Pulse,** and **If the Child Is Vomiting or Is Bleeding From the Mouth,** pages 49–50.
- **Don't** bend the child's neck or twist his or her body if her or she is unconscious or if a back or neck injury is suspected. See **Back and Neck Injuries,** page 45.
- **Don't** try to clean foreign matter from a deep scalp wound.
- **Don't** give the child pain relievers without first consulting the child's doctor.

- If, after consulting these pages, you have determined that the head injury is minor, refer to **Home Treatment,** page 150.

If the Child is Unconscious (Not Responsive)

If the child is unconscious, assume there is a back or neck injury. Handle the child carefully. Do not bend or twist his body or neck.

1. Check the child for signs of a head injury, as follows:

- Breathing
  The breathing pattern is irregular—the child may take several breaths, followed by several seconds of no breathing. Breaths may be very deep and/or very slow. The child may have difficulty breathing. If the child is not breathing, see **Rescue Breathing/ Cardiopulmonary Resuscitation (CPR),** immediately: 0–1 year, page 27; 1–8 years, page 33; 8+ years, page 39.
- Outward signs
  Clear fluid or blood is draining from the ears, nose, and/or mouth. There is a skull deformity —a swollen area or a sunken area on the head. There is a head wound or a bruise on the head. The child has black eyes or blackness behind the ears (may take hours to days to appear).
- Neurological changes
  The child has a seizure. The child has no response or varied responses to pain. (Pinch different parts of the child's body—some body parts may react; some may not.)

- Signs of shock
  The child has cold, moist skin; pale skin, becoming purplish; pale or bluish lips, nails, or gums; rapid pulse; weakness; and/or restlessness. Signs may not appear immediately.
- Gastrointestinal signs
  The child is vomiting.

2. Prevent the child's head from moving.

a. Keep the child's head in the same position in which you found it.

b. Place rolled-up clothing, blankets, or whatever else is available, around the child's head and neck. Keep them in place with books, stones, or other heavy objects. (Figures 3, 4)

3. Keep the airway clear.

a. Clear the child's mouth of blood and tooth or bone fragments.

b. If the child vomits, carefully turn him onto his side while supporting his head and keeping his head in line with his body. Do not just turn his head. See **Back and Neck Injuries: If the Child Is Vomiting or Is Bleeding From the Mouth,** page 50.

4. Monitor the child's breathing and pulse.

a. Observe the child's breathing. If there is difficulty breathing, keep his head in position to keep the airway open. If there is a possibility of a back or neck injury, do not bend the child's neck or tilt his head back. Place two or three fingers under each side of his lower jaw and lift upward (jaw-thrust technique). (Figure 5)

Figure 3

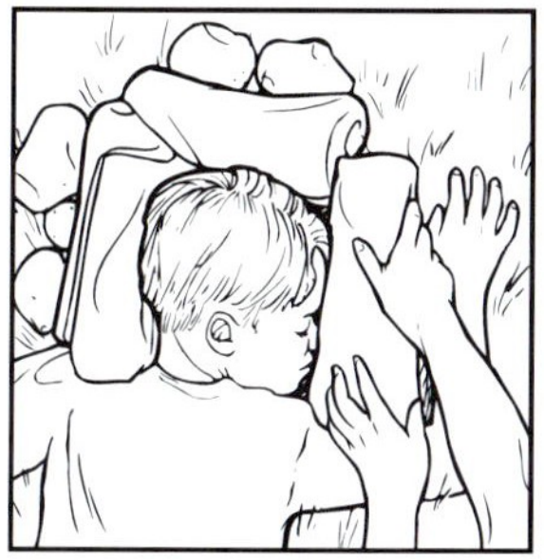

Figure 4

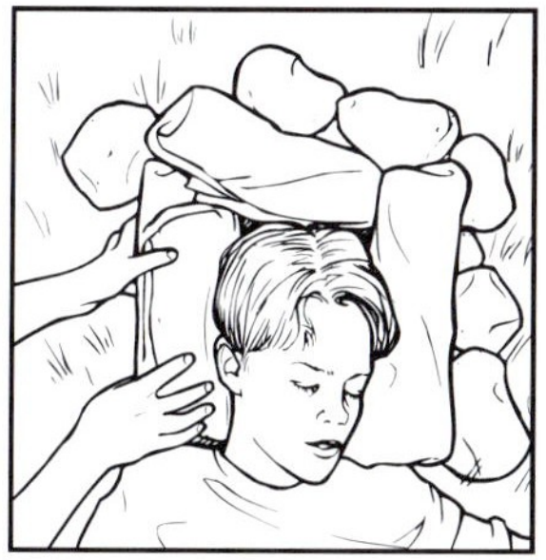

Figure 5

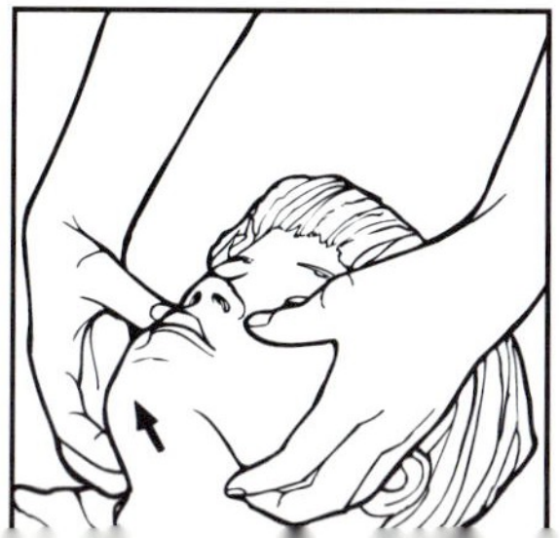

b. If breathing stops, begin rescue breathing. See **Rescue Breathing/Cardiopulmonary Resuscitation (CPR):** 0–1 year, page 27; 1–8 years, page 33; 8+ years, page 39.

c. If the pulse stops, begin cardiopulmonary resuscitation. See **Rescue Breathing/ Cardiopulmonary Resuscitation (CPR):** 0–1 year, page 27; 1–8 years, page 33; 8+ years, page 39.

If the Child Is Conscious (Awake)

1. Check the child for signs of a serious head injury, as follows:

- Breathing
  The breathing pattern is irregular—the child may take several breaths, followed by several seconds of no breathing. Breaths may be very deep and/or very slow. The child may have difficulty breathing.
- Outward signs
  Clear fluid or blood is draining from the ears, nose, and/or mouth. There is a skull deformity—a swollen area or a sunken area on the head. There is a head wound or a bruise on the head. The child has black eyes or blackness behind the ears (may take hours to days to appear).
- Altered level of consciousness
  The child cannot answer simple age-appropriate questions, such as questions about his name, age, or siblings' names. The child is confused and/or drowsy.
- Neurological changes
  The child has a seizure. The child is unable to move one or more parts of his body. The child has blurred vision. The child's pulse is slow. (See **Range of Normal Heart Rates at Rest,** page 13.)

3. Keep the child lying down.

a. If there is no sign of a back or neck injury (see **Back and Neck Injuries,** page 45), raise the child's head and shoulders and place a pillow, clothing, or whatever else is available behind his head and shoulders so it comes down to the middle of his back. Avoid pressure on the back of the child's neck. (Figure 6)

b. Apply ice wrapped in plastic or cloth if there is any swelling.

Figure 6

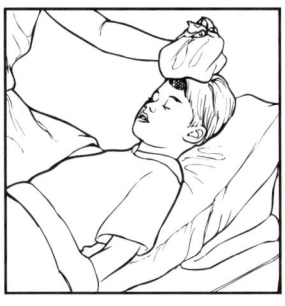

4. Watch the child's breathing.

a. Clear the child's mouth of blood and tooth or bone fragments.

b. Observe the child for signs of breathing difficulty. If signs develop, sit the child in a more upright position, supporting his head, shoulders, and back. **Call 911 or the rescue squad.** See **Breathing Difficulty—General,** page 71.

c. If the child stops breathing, see **Rescue Breathing/Cardiopulmonary Resuscitation (CPR):** 0–1 year, page 27; 1–8 years, page 33; 8+ years, page 39.

When to See a Doctor

Call the child's doctor to report the incident. Describe all signs, and follow the doctor's recommendations. Take the child to see a doctor if any of the following apply:

- The child develops any variation of these signs within hours or days of the accident: inability to awaken from sleep, weakness, continuous drowsiness, slurred speech, changes in vision, uncoordinated movements, or continuous vomiting.
- The child has a deep, wide, or large scalp or face wound, or foreign matter is deeply embedded in the wound.
- Signs of a wound infection develop—thick, yellow or green drainage; foul odor; redness; hardened wound edges; or fever.

Home Treatment

Children often hit their heads on furniture or fall a short distance, such as from a chair. If the child does not have signs of a more serious head injury, as previously described, do the following:

1. Control bleeding with sterile gauze or clean cloths applied lightly to the wound. If the wound is deep, large, or wide, bandage the dressing in place and have the wound examined by a doctor. For minor cuts only, gently wash the cut with soap and water and reapply the dressing. Change the dressing daily and when soiled or wet.
2. Apply ice to a bump on the head to prevent swelling.
3. Avoid medications to relieve immediate headache or vomiting; they may cover up important signs of serious injury.

4. If the injury was caused by force (a hit) or by impact with an object (perhaps the child fell down the stairs or walked into a door), check every 2 hours for:
   - Breathing—much shallower and faster or much deeper and slower than usual (See **Range of Normal Breathing Rates at Rest,** page 15.)
   - Pulse—very slow (0–1 year—less than 80 beats per minute; 1+ years—less than 60 beats per minute) (See **Range of Normal Heart Rates at Rest,** page 13.)
   - Difficulty awakening the child
   - Signs of shock (See **Shock,** page 169.)

   If all signs are normal, you may allow the child to rest. However, report any suspicious signs to the doctor immediately.
5. Ask the doctor if it is all right to use acetaminophen to relieve any headache that is still present a few days after the injury.
6. Inform the doctor of any personality changes, such as moodiness and irritability, that the child experiences in the days or weeks following the injury.

Safety Highlights

Do

- **Do** call the Poison Control Center or the child's doctor immediately.
- **Do** save the product container and any available samples of the pills, powder, or liquid that the child ingested, for examination.
- **Do** save a sample of the child's vomit, if available, for examination.

Don't

- **Don't** give the child anything to drink if he or she is unconscious.
- **Don't** rely on poison instructions on a product label; they may be out of date.
- **Don't** wait for symptoms to appear—if you suspect poisoning, call the Poison Control Center immediately.

Immediate Action

1. Look at the surroundings and the general appearance of the child.

(Take a few seconds.) (Figure 1)

- Is there an open container near the child or in an area where the child may have been?
- Are there pieces of pills, drops of liquid, or spilled powder or crystals near the child?
- Is there evidence of a substance in or around the child's mouth or on his hands or clothing? If so, note the color, odor, and consistency (powdery, gooey, oily, and so on).
- Are there burns around the child's mouth?

If the answer to any of the above is *yes,* the child may have swallowed a poisonous substance.

Figure 1

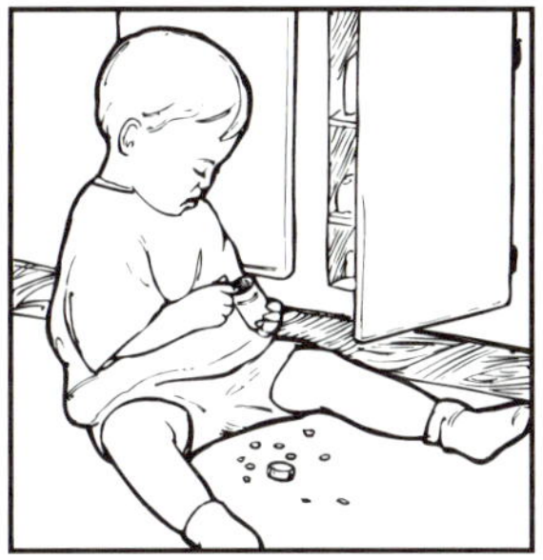

2. Check for and treat the most life-threatening problems now.

Check for signs of unconsciousness, no breathing, no pulse, bleeding, and shock. (Figure 2) See **Life-Threat Checklist,** page 23. **Call 911 or the rescue squad** as recommended in **Life-Threat Checklist.**

Once the most life-threatening problems have been attended to, you may proceed with further treatment as instructed below.

Figure 2

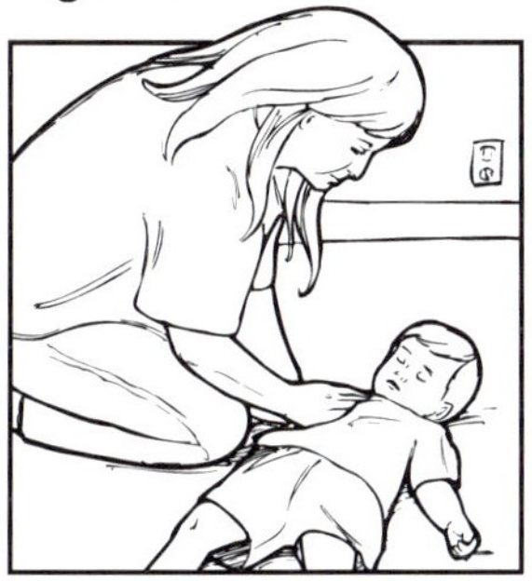

3. Check the child for signs of poisoning:

- Abdominal pain, nausea, vomiting
- Drowsiness or difficulty in awakening from sleep
- Slow breathing rate (See **Checking Respiration (Breathing),** page 14.)
- Slow pulse (See **Checking Pulse,** page 13.)
- Unconsciousness (no response when the child is shaken gently or his name is called loudly)
- Seizure (See **Seizures,** page 165.)
- Slurred speech
- Lack of coordination

4. If the child is experiencing a slow breathing rate, slow pulse, unconsciousness, or seizures, call 911 or the rescue squad.

5. If poisoning is suspected, call the Poison Control Center.

Phone #______________________________

If there is no Poison Control Center in your area, call the child's doctor,

Phone #______________________________

OR

the local hospital emergency department.

Phone #________________________________

If available, bring the poison container to the phone. (Figure 3)

a. Make the phone call as soon as you suspect the child has swallowed a poison. Do not wait for symptoms to appear.

b. Describe the child's symptoms.

c. Name or describe the substance swallowed and estimate the quantity swallowed.

d. Write down and follow the instructions you are given.

If you cannot reach medical assistance by telephone, follow the instructions in Step 7, page 156.

6. Stimulate vomiting if you are instructed to do so.

If the child is awake and alert, and the Poison Control Center, doctor, or hospital emergency personnel instruct you to do so, stimulate vomiting.

NOTE: *Many substances should not be vomited as they will burn the child's esophagus (food tube), throat, and mouth as they come up. Stimulate vomiting only upon medical advice.*

a. Give the child syrup of ipecac (available at most drugstores). (Figure 4) If syrup of ipecac is unavailable, proceed to Step e.

b. Follow syrup of ipecac with one or two glasses of warm water. (Figure 5)

c. Have the child vomit into a bucket or bowl and retain this sample to bring to the medical facility.

d. If there is no vomiting within 30 minutes, repeat Steps a and b.

Figure 3

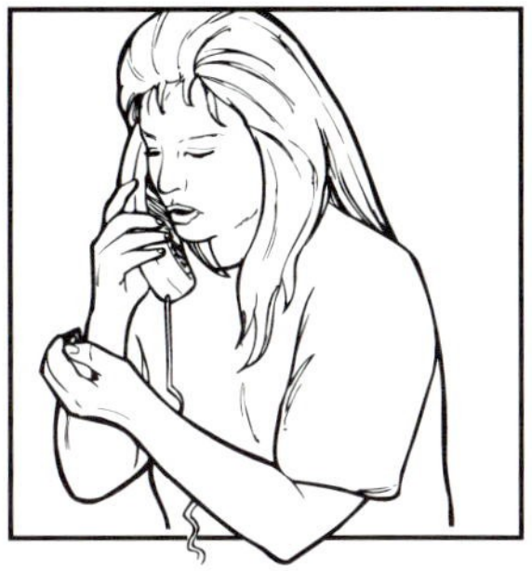

Syrup of Ipecac Dosage Chart	
0–1 year	2 teaspoons
1–8 years	1 tablespoon
9+ years	2 tablespoons

Figure 4

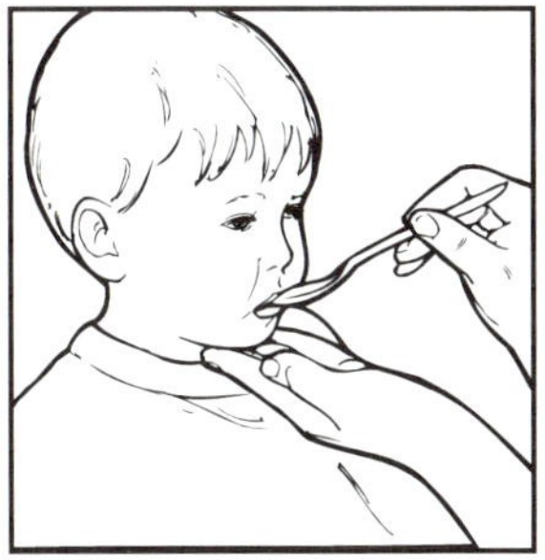

Figure 5

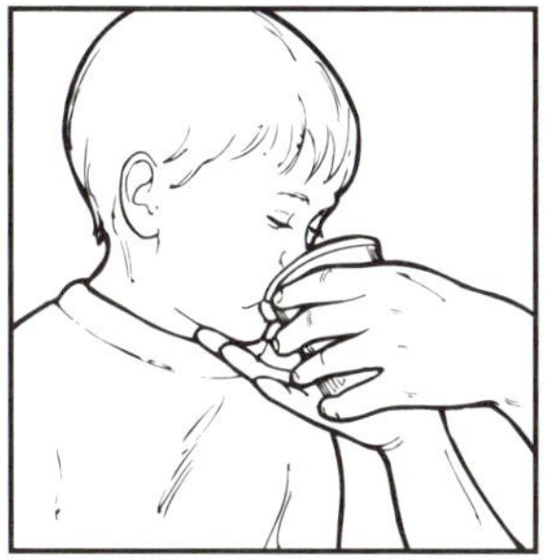

When to See a Doctor

Take the child to see a doctor if either of the following applies:

- You are instructed to do so by the Poison Control Center, the doctor, or the hospital emergency personnel.
- There is not a Poison Control Center in your area, the child's doctor and the local hospital emergency department are not available by phone, and you know or suspect that the child has swallowed a poisonous substance.

Home Treatment

Treat the child as directed by the Poison Control Center or the doctor.

Safety Highlights

Do

- **Do** perform all movements carefully to prevent the object that caused the wound from moving.
- **Do** apply a bandage tightly enough to stabilize the object that caused the wound, but loosen it if the limb becomes cold, blue, or numb.

Don't

- **Don't** move or remove the object that caused the wound.
- **Don't** move the child off an impaling object unless you must do so to protect the child from danger.
- **Don't** use iodine, merbromin (for example, Mercurochrome®), or other antiseptics on the wound without first checking with the doctor.

Immediate Action

1. Look at the surroundings and the general appearance of the child.

(Take a few seconds.)

- Did the child fall onto an object that pierced through a part of her body (impaled her) *and* is the child's life endangered by her location? (For example, is there an electrical rod involved?) If the answer is *yes,* carefully move the child off the object. If the child's life is not in danger, do not move her.
- Does the child have an object sticking out of a part of her body? (Figure 1) If the answer is *yes,* do not move the object.

Figure 1

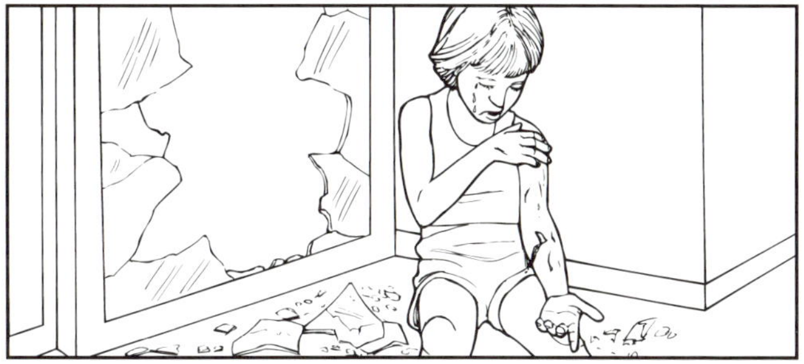

4. Stabilize the object that caused the wound.

a. Cut any clothing away from around the wound.

b. Apply layers of sterile gauze or clean cloths around the object to make a bulky dressing. (Figure 5)

c. Hold the dressing and the object in place by wrapping strips of cloth around the dressing and the injured body part. You should be able to slide a finger beneath the dressing. (Figure 6)

d. If an arm or leg is involved, stabilize them against the body. (See **Splinting Techniques,** pages 134–140.)

e. If the protruding object is very long, carefully cut the object at a point several inches away from its point of entry. (Figure 7)

5. Seek medical assistance.

a. Call 911 or the rescue squad if:

- Bleeding cannot be controlled.
- The child is having difficulty breathing. See **Breathing Difficulty—General,** page 71. If the child stops breathing, see **Rescue Breathing/Cardiopulmonary Resuscitation (CPR):** 0–1 year, page 27; 1–8 years, page 33; 8+ years, page 39.

b. Transport the child to a medical facility as long as:

- Bleeding has been controlled, and
- The child is not having breathing difficulty.

Figure 5

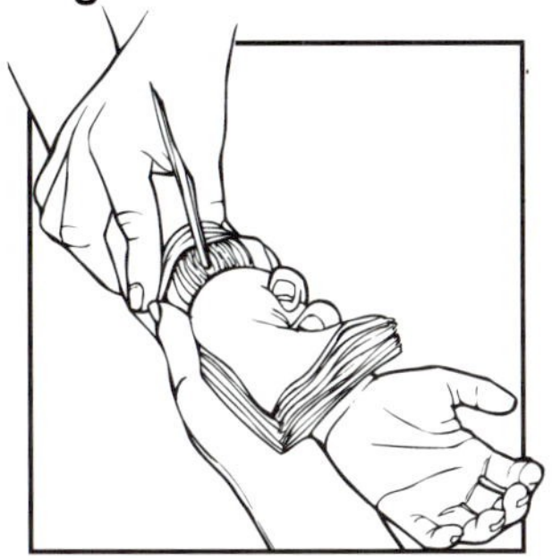

Figure 6

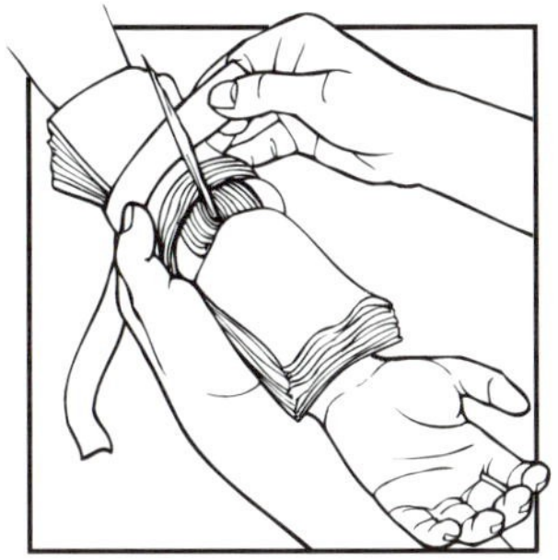

Figure 7

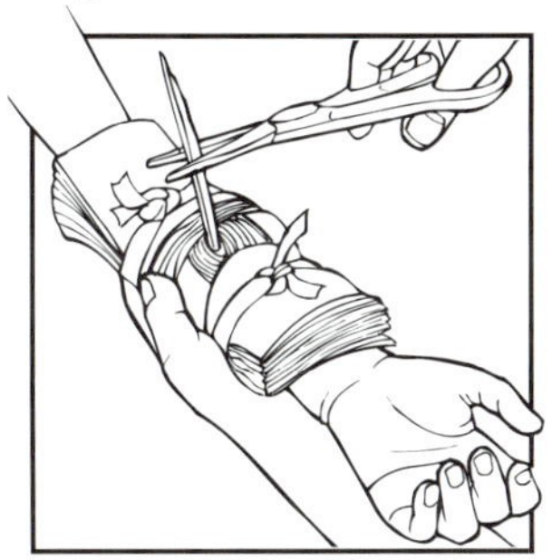

6. While awaiting medical help or on the way to the medical facility, observe the child for life-threatening problems.

a. Observe the child's breathing. Be sure the child's head is properly positioned for an open airway. (Figure 8) If breathing stops, begin rescue breathing. See **Rescue Breathing/ Cardiopulmonary Resuscitation (CPR):** 0–1 year, page 27; 1–8 years, page 33; 8+ years, page 39.

b. Observe the child's level of consciousness. If the child becomes unconscious, see **Rescue Breathing/ Cardiopulmonary Resuscitation (CPR):** 0–1 year, page 27; 1–8 years, page 33; 8+ years, page 39.

c. Observe and treat for shock. See **Shock,** page 169.

Figure 8

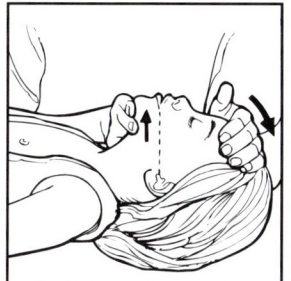

When to See a Doctor

Take the child to see a doctor if any of the following apply:

- The object, part of the object, or other foreign matter remains in the wound.
- There is numbness or tingling around or beyond the wound.
- The child has not had a tetanus shot within five years.
- The impaling object was rusty or dirty.
- Signs of wound infection develop—thick, yellow or green drainage; swelling; redness and hardening around the puncture site; pain at the site; or fever.

Home Treatment

A doctor may not be needed for minor puncture wounds. If none of the items listed in **When to See a Doctor,** above, apply and if bleeding has been controlled, do the following:

1. Wash the wound with soap and water. A solution of half-strength hydrogen peroxide may be applied to the wound. (Pour a small amount of hydrogen peroxide into a cup, and add an equal amount of water.)
2. Check the wound for part of the impaling object or other foreign matter. See a doctor if the object or other foreign matter remains in the wound.
3. Apply a dry, sterile-gauze dressing to keep the wound clean. Change the dressing daily and if it becomes soiled or wet.
4. Soak the wound in warm water for fifteen minutes three to four times a day for the next 4–5 days; reapply a dry dressing after soaking.
5. Check the wound daily for signs of infection, and notify the doctor if they occur.

Safety Highlights

Do

- **Do** clear the area of objects that may injure the child having a seizure.
- **Do** note the times at which the seizure began and ended. (Most seizures from a fever last 2–3 minutes.)
- **Do** keep the child's airway open during the seizure.
- **Do** begin fever-reducing measures immediately after the seizure has ended, if the child has a fever.

Don't

- **Don't** put anything into the child's mouth during the seizure.
- **Don't** try to hold the child still during the seizure.
- **Don't** give the child anything to drink if he or she is very drowsy after the seizure.
- **Don't** put a thermometer in the child's mouth if he or she is drowsy; take a rectal temperature instead.

Immediate Action

1. Look at the child for signs of a seizure:

- Falling to the floor
- Eyes rolling upward or to the side
- Stiffening of the body
- Violent jerking movements of the arms and/or legs that may involve only one side of the body (Movements are continuous and rhythmic.)
- Pale or blue tinge to the lips, nails, gums, or skin around the mouth
- Drooling and foaming at the mouth
- Arching of the back

2. Note the time the seizure began.

The length of most seizures ranges from several seconds to several minutes.

3. Protect the child from injury.

a. Move hard objects away from the child.

b. Move the child away from walls and furniture.

c. Do not hold the child down.

d. Place pillows, blankets, or rolled-up clothing around the child. (Figure 1)

4. Maintain an open airway.

a. Do not force any object into the child's mouth.

b. Observe the child and assist with open-airway maintenance as necessary. If breathing is very noisy or color is becoming pale with blue-tinged lips, gums, or nails, gently tilt the child's head back, with one hand lifting her chin and the other hand on her forehead. This should straighten and open the airway. Hold the child's head in this position. (Figure 2) See airway-opening technique in **Rescue Breathing/Cardiopulmonary Resuscitation (CPR):** 0–1 year, page 27; 1–8 years, page 33; 8+ years, page 39.

5. Note the time the seizure ends.

Call 911 or the rescue squad if the seizure lasts more than 3 minutes.

After a seizure, the child may be very drowsy, may vomit, may urinate or have a bowel movement.

Figure 1

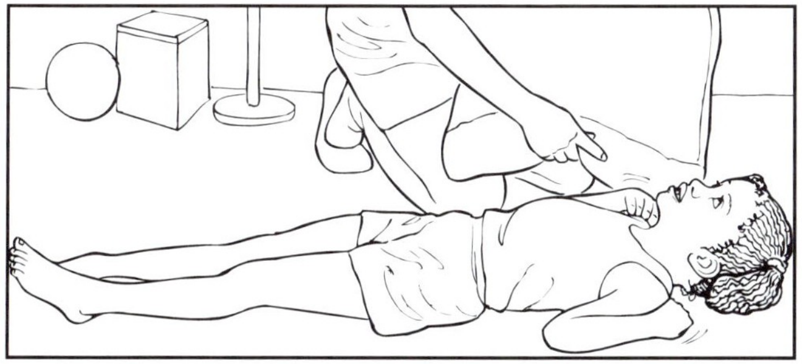

Figure 2

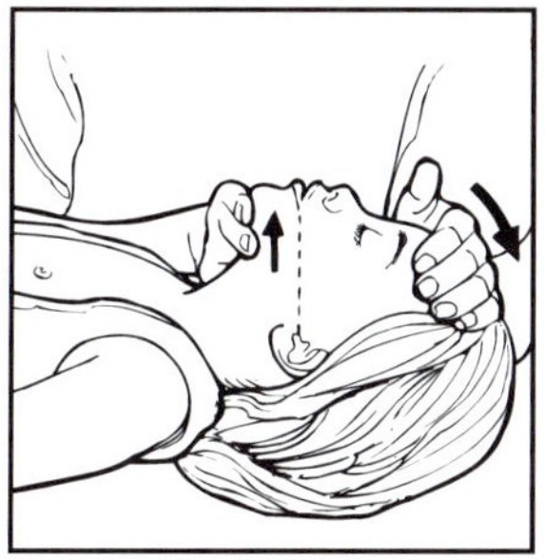

6. Observe the child after the seizure.

a. Maintain an open airway.

b. Look, listen, and feel for breathing. (Figure 3)

c. If the child is not breathing, have someone **call 911 or the rescue squad.** Begin rescue breathing. See **Rescue Breathing/ Cardiopulmonary Resuscitation (CPR):** 0–1 year, page 27; 1–8 years, page 33; 8+ years, page 39.

d. If the child is breathing but remains very drowsy, turn her onto her side to allow fluids to drain from her mouth. (Figure 4) Keep her head straight—her chin should not be touching her chest.

e. If the child vomits, clear her mouth and keep her on her side.

f. If the child has never had a seizure before, this episode may be due to a fever. In some children, a rapid rise in temperature, usually to over 102°F, can cause a seizure. This is most common in children 6 months to 6 years of age. Take the child's temperature. (See **Checking Temperature,** page 16.) If temperature is elevated, see **Fever,** page 125.

g. If the child has a history of seizures for which she is being treated by a doctor, follow the instructions previously given to you by the doctor.

h. If the child has another seizure within an hour, **call 911 or the rescue squad.**

7. Call the child's doctor.

Report the episode to the child's doctor and follow the doctor's instructions. The child may have to be examined by the doctor, especially if this is the child's first seizure, and anti-seizure medications may be in order.

Figure 3

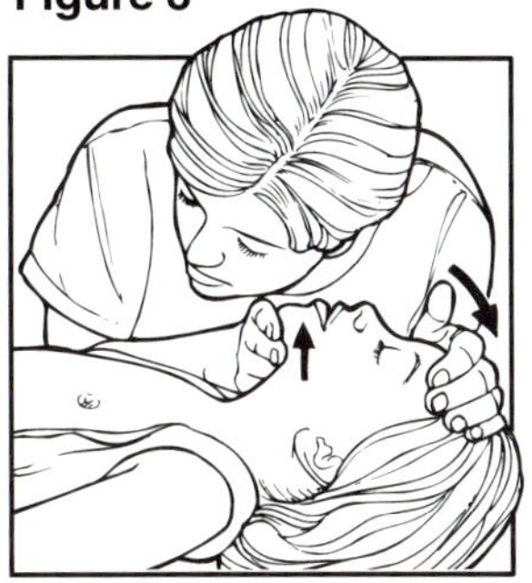

Figure 4

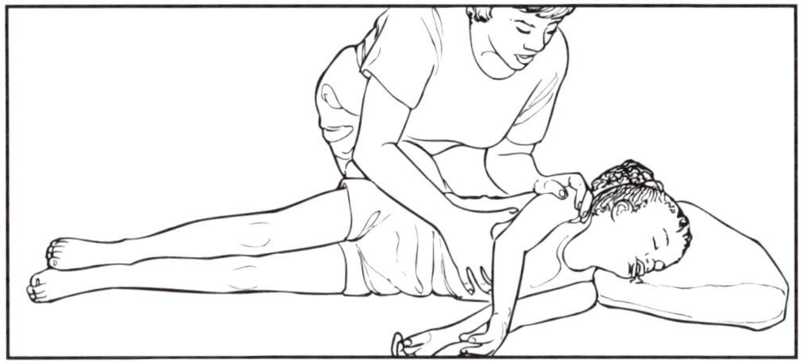

SEIZURES

Shock is a condition in which blood pressure is so low that blood cannot reach the brain and other organs rapidly enough and in amounts necessary for them to function properly. Shock must be treated promptly to prevent organ failure and death.

Causes of shock include the following: large loss of blood or other fluids (internal or external); severe burns; serious infection; poisoning; drug overdose; insulin shock, for those suffering from diabetes; heart attack; allergic reaction to medication, food, an insect or animal bite, or environmental allergens; lack of oxygen; severe spinal cord injury; and traumatic emotional events.

Safety Highlights

Do

- **Do** be prepared to give the doctor as much information as possible about the cause of shock. (For example, was the child exposed to something that he or she is allergic to? Did the child suffer a serious injury? Is the child a diabetic?)
- **Do** have another person control bleeding if you are performing rescue breathing or cardiopulmonary resuscitation (CPR).

Don't

- **Don't** move the child if a back or neck injury is suspected.
- **Don't** move the child if he or she is unconscious and a head injury is suspected.
- **Don't** give the child anything to eat or drink.
- **Don't** leave the child alone, except to call for medical assistance, as directed.

Immediate Action

1. Look at the surroundings and the general appearance of the child.

(Take a few seconds.)

- Has the child been seriously injured? (Perhaps she was thrown from a vehicle, suffered a major fall, suffered a severe wound resulting in a large amount of bleeding, or suffered serious burns over a large part of her body.) (Figure 1)
- Was the child exposed to something to which she is severely allergic, such as a bee sting, food, or medication?
- Is there evidence of ingestion of a poison or of a drug overdose?
- Does the child have a history of diabetes?
- Was the child without oxygen due to suffocation, drowning, smoke inhalation, or some other cause?
- Did the child have a severe emotional reaction to a stressful event?

If the answer to any of the above is *yes,* the child is at risk for developing shock.

2. Check for signs of shock:

- Cold, moist skin
- Rapid, faint pulse (See **Checking Pulse,** page 13.)
- Pale skin; may become purplish
- Pale or blue lips, gums, or nails
- Weak, rapid, and shallow breathing pattern, or breathing may be deep but irregular and/or the child may be gasping
- Unconsciousness (no response when you gently shake the child's shoulder or call her name loudly)

Figure 1

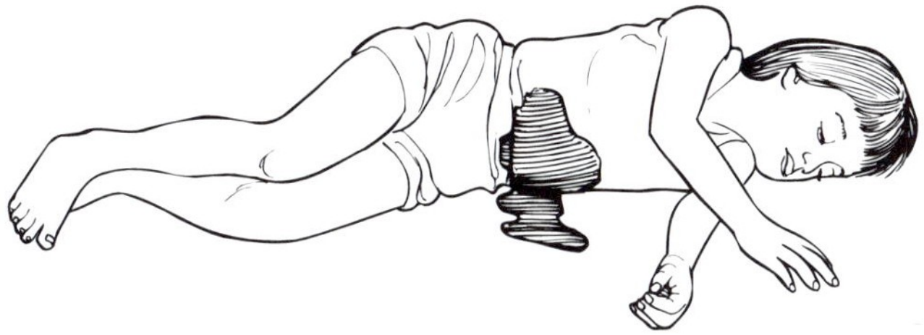

- Weakness, possible fainting
- Restlessness, anxiety
- Extreme thirst
- Nausea

3. If shock is suspected, seek medical assistance.

Call 911 or the rescue squad. While awaiting medical assistance, proceed to Step 4.

4. Check for and treat the most life-threatening problems now.

Check for signs of unconsciousness, no breathing, no pulse, and bleeding. (Figure 2)

- If the child is unconscious, not breathing, or has no pulse, see **Rescue Breathing/Cardiopulmonary Resuscitation (CPR):** 0–1 year, page 27; 1–8 years, page 33; 8+ years, page 39.
- If the child has breathing difficulty, see **Breathing Difficulty—General,** page 71.
- If the child is bleeding, see **Bleeding and Cuts,** page 63.

5. Position the child.

Find the appropriate position for the child based on the criteria below.

Leave the child in the position in which you found her if:

- you suspect a back or neck injury but the child is conscious and breathing.

NOTE: *Suspect a back or neck injury if the child is unconscious and there was a severe blow to the head, or if the child's body or neck was twisted or forced backward violently. Do not bend or twist the child's body. If you must move the child, support her head*

Figure 2

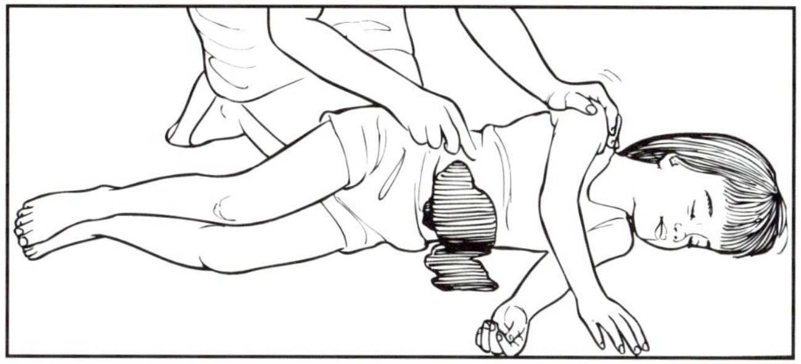

7. Prevent heat loss.

a. Put one or more blankets under the child, but do not move the child to do so if you suspect a back or neck injury.

b. Cover the child with a blanket, clothing, or something else for warmth. However, if the environment is very hot, do not cover the child. (Figure 5)

Figure 5

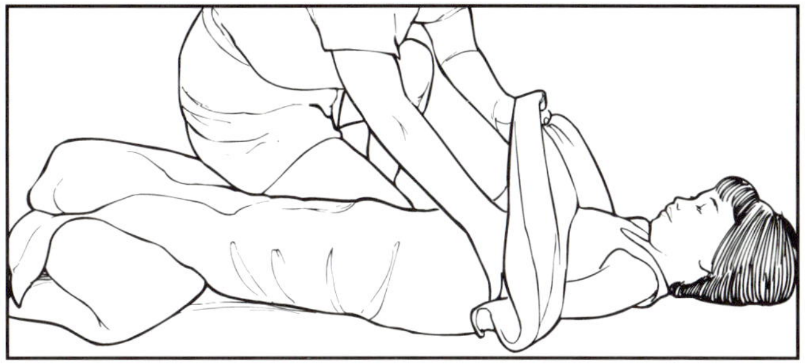

8. Splint suspected fractures.

See **Fractures (Broken Bones) and Sprains,** page 129, for symptoms of a fracture and splinting techniques to hold the injured part still. Movement of the part can cause more bleeding.

9. Observe the child.

a. Continue to observe breathing. If the child develops difficulty breathing, she is conscious, and you do not suspect a back or neck injury, raise her head and shoulders. (Figure 6) If she stops breathing, begin rescue breathing. See **Rescue Breathing/ Cardiopulmonary Resuscitation (CPR):** 0–1 year, page 27; 1–8 years, page 33; 8+ years, page 39.

b. Check the child's pulse. If pulse stops, begin cardiopulmonary resuscitation. See **Rescue Breathing/Cardiopulmonary Resuscitation (CPR):** 0–1 year, page 27; 1–8 years, page 33; 8+ years, page 39.

c. Keep the child lying still.

d. Do not give the child anything to eat or drink. If the child needs emergency surgery, her stomach should be empty.

Figure 6

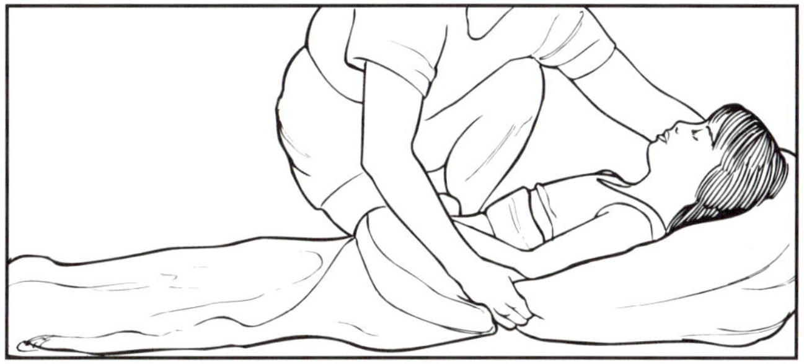

When to See a Doctor

All children with symptoms of shock must be seen by a doctor, preferably in a hospital equipped to handle such an emergency. The child should be transported by ambulance.

Home Treatment

Shock is a medical emergency that must be attended to by a doctor.

Many children have behavioral disturbances during and following hospitalization—even brief hospitalization for relatively minor treatment. A hospital experience can be stressful for anyone for three distinct reasons: separation from parents and/or significant others, loss of control, and subjection to painful and/or intrusive procedures. Hospitalization is particularly stressful for children because it involves change—that is, change in their usual state of health and in their daily routine—and because children have limited coping mechanisms. A child's understanding of, reaction to, and method of coping with hospitalization are influenced by the child's age and stage of development; his or her past experience with hospitalization, illness, injury, or separation; his or her support system (family, peers, and so on); and the severity of the illness or injury. The following material summarizes, for different age groups, the causes of stress (stressors), the behavioral reactions you can expect, and ways you can help the child cope with the hospital experience.

Infants (0–1 Year)

Stressors	Behavioral reactions
Separation (more pronounced after 4 months of age)	Protest: The infant cries and screams, searches for the parent or caregiver with his eyes, clings to the parent, and avoids and rejects contact with strangers. Despair: The infant is withdrawn, depressed, and uninterested in his environment.
Pain	Before 6 months of age, infants do not appear to remember past painful experiences, and therefore are not apprehensive about future experiences. They react to pain with bodily movements and loud crying but can be distracted easily. After 6 months of age, infants can anticipate pain and may react by struggling and trying to resist medical procedures.
Immobilization	The infant cries, is irritable, and experiences a disturbed sleep pattern.

Loss of control (physical restriction, loss of routine and rituals)	The toddler may display resistance; physical aggression; uncooperativeness; regression to earlier forms of behavior (demands a bottle after she has been weaned, wants others to feed her, refuses to use the toilet); and negativism, especially in the form of temper tantrums. Later, the child may withdraw, preferring not to interact with others.
Bodily injury and pain	The child may react intensely to procedures that are intrusive, such as a hospital staff member taking her temperature or blood pressure, examining her ears, giving her oral medications, and so on. Although these procedures are not painful, the child views them as things "being done to her" that are out of her control and therefore very threatening. The child may physically resist, cry loudly, run away, or cling to the parent or caregiver for protection. The toddler is able to remember painful experiences. If she is exposed to a painful procedure more than once, the toddler will often react with extreme emotional upset, physical resistance, and loud crying or will retreat to the parent or caregiver. The child's reaction will be influenced by whether there is a separation from parents or caregivers, the degree of physical restraint, past experiences, and the degree of preparation for a procedure.

Coping Strategies

Ask the hospital staff if you can be with the child during medical procedures. If you are allowed to be present, give emotional support to the child by holding her hand or verbally encouraging her. If the procedure is not a painful one, you may be able to hold the child on your lap. Do not try to assist with the procedure, however, especially if it is a painful one. The child looks to you for comfort, security, and protection. Your involvement in hurting her will confuse her and weaken her trust in you. Your role should be to comfort the child during and after procedures.

MEETING EMOTIONAL NEEDS

If the child must be admitted to the hospital, at least one parent should try to be with the child as much as possible. Many hospitals have sleeping accommodations for a parent in the child's room, excluding intensive-care units. If the child's condition allows, a parent may be able to perform routine care, such as bathing, feeding, and rocking.

Bring one or two of the child's favorite toys or a favorite blanket to the hospital. Place a photograph of the child's family where she can see it. Plan appropriate activities for the child, depending on her condition and the restrictions on her activities ordered by the doctor. To make the hospital seem more like home, parents should try to carry out as many routine activities with the child as possible. The child's condition will limit some of these activities, but reading at bedtime, taking a bottle at certain times of the day, brushing teeth after meals, saying prayers, and so on may still be possible. Do not expect the child to succeed at performing newly learned skills, however. If the child is in the process of becoming toilet trained, for example, she may have more "accidents" than usual in the hospital. Toilet training can be resumed when the child returns home.

Prepare the child for medical procedures. The hospital staff member performing a procedure should explain what he or she is going to do in simple language. You might give further explanation by relating the procedure to another experience familiar to the child. For example, you might say, "Remember, you had this medicine before and it tasted very good," or, "Remember, I took your temperature before and it didn't hurt." Most importantly, be honest with the child. If she has to have a needle inserted to receive fluids, for example, admit to her that it will hurt a little bit but that the hurt will not last very long and that afterward she can have a special reward (a special television show, a special toy, and so on). The staff member may be able to demonstrate the procedure first on a doll, on another toy, or on you. This will be comforting to the child.

The child may want a parent or caregiver near her as much as possible after discharge from the hospital. Plan to spend extra time with the child to allow her to feel secure again.

Preschoolers (3–6 Years)

Stressors	Behavioral reactions
Separation	Normally, the preschooler can tolerate brief periods of separation from parents and can develop trust in other significant adults. However, he has difficulty coping with parental separation when faced with the stress of hospitalization. He may protest the separation and demonstrate his anxiety by refusing to eat, withdrawing from interaction with others, crying quietly for his parents, having difficulty sleeping, or continually asking for his parents. The child may show his anger by playing more aggressively, breaking his toys, hitting other children, or refusing to cooperate in performing routine care, such as brushing his teeth. Both boys and girls of preschool age begin to have a closer relationship with their fathers than they did at earlier stages of development. Preschoolers may prefer the presence of their fathers when stressed by hospitalization, and mothers should understand that this is a normal stage of development. Later, the child may withdraw from contact with others and show anger to his parents for having left him.
Loss of control (physical restriction, loss of routine and rituals)	The preschooler normally views himself as all-powerful. He uses "magical thinking" to believe that he is capable of doing whatever he imagines. His fantasy view of the world may lead him to develop bizarre explanations for events, especially when he is faced with an unfamiliar experience (in this case, a loss of routine due to hospitalization). An injured child may imagine that he was

act brave as a result. However, this age group also understands the benefits of being sick. They know that complaints of pain bring attention, and therefore such complaints must be evaluated by parents and caregivers in the context of other symptoms and other stressful events, such as the birth of a sibling or the beginning of kindergarten.

Preschoolers react to anticipated pain in several different ways. Some children use aggression; they may try to push away the person they view as inflicting pain on them or they may grab equipment and refuse to have it "used on them." Other children may run and hide. Some children may verbalize their apprehension, with expressions such as "Go away" or "I hate you." If a child views a medical procedure as punishment, he may try to bargain, with expressions such as "I'll be good; please don't give me that shot." The child may also cry and shout during the procedure, saying, "No, stop, it hurts." The child reacts to a procedure in this manner even if the procedure is not particularly painful because he fears the unknown, he is confused about why someone is hurting him, and he is anxious about being restrained for the procedure.

It is common for a preschool child to resort to dependent behavior when faced with a stressful event. The fear of pain or separation may cause the child to cling to the parent or caregiver and want to be held continuously. The child may not want to be left alone and may either cry for the parent or caregiver if he or she must leave, or become withdrawn, refusing to play with other children or interact with hospital staff members. The child may also revert to an earlier stage of development, requiring assistance with skills that have already been learned, such as dressing or bathing.

Some children react to pain or other stress with bodily responses such as breathing very rapidly, becoming very restless, or vomiting.

Coping Strategies

Ask the hospital staff if you can be with the child during medical procedures. If you are allowed to be present, give emotional support to the child by holding his hand or by verbally encouraging him. Do not try to assist with the procedure, however, especially if it is a painful one. The child looks to you for comfort, security, and protection. Your involvement in hurting him will confuse him and weaken his trust in you. Your role should be to comfort the child during and after procedures.

If the child must be admitted to the hospital, at least one parent should try to be with the child as much as possible. Many hospitals have sleeping accommodations for a parent in the child's room, excluding intensive-care units. If the child's condition allows, a parent may be able to perform routine care, such as bathing and feeding. Bring one or two of the child's favorite toys or books to the hospital.

Encourage the child to talk about his fears and expectations. Clarify any misunderstandings he has with honest explanations of what has happened and what will have to be done for him to get better. Use terms the child can understand and use pictures or dolls to increase his understanding. Reassure the child that he did not do anything bad to cause his illness or injury and that he is not being punished. If a child's injury actually was a direct result of disobedience, this is not the time to scold the child. He needs support and reassurance to help him cope with the present situation.

Allow the child to act out his feelings in play. He may want to give a doll a "shot" to "get back" at the nurse who gave him an injection and thus regain a feeling of control. If possible, allow the child to handle a surgical mask and gloves, a medicine cup, a blood pressure cuff, or a stethoscope to reduce his fear of these unfamiliar items.

Address the child's nurses, doctors, and therapists by name and explain their roles, to help the child perceive them as familiar people rather than as strangers intent on hurting him.

As the child's condition improves, he should be allowed to have more control over his environment. Let the child choose foods to eat from those allowed on his diet and let him decide on which books to read. Tell the child in advance about procedures that will occur. Treat routine, painless procedures casually, like a game that the child will take part in. His participation will help him feel more control over his environment.

When faced with an emergency procedure, there may be little time to prepare the child. If permitted, try to stay close enough during the procedure for the child to see or at least hear you. Talk soothingly to him, reassuring him that he will be okay. Remain calm to prevent added anxiety in the child. Comfort the child after the procedure and explain the events to him in words he can understand. If there is time before a procedure, prepare the child with an honest description of what to expect, but do it in simple terms and without too many details that may confuse or scare him. Relate explanations to other situations with which he is familiar. For example, you might say, "Remember when Danny had a cast on his leg?" Be honest about describing the degree of pain to expect. You might say, "Yes, it will hurt a little when the nurse puts your IV in, but only for a minute. Then she'll tape it on and it will feel okay. See the other kids? They have IVs and they can still play." Emphasize the positive rather than the negative; avoid over-sympathizing. Ask hospital staff members to explain procedures to the child if you are unfamiliar with them.

If the child is facing surgery, it may be helpful to show him the body part that will be involved and to use the term "fix it" to explain what is going to be done. Tell the

	Feelings of loneliness, boredom, isolation, and depression may occur. Some children may become quiet and withdrawn. They still need adult guidance and support but may be afraid to ask for it, for fear of appearing weak and dependent. Unable to express their negative feelings verbally, they may express such feelings through hostile or aggressive behavior, irritability, or rejection of siblings. The older school-age child may prefer not to have the continued presence of a parent at the hospital because she is trying to assert her independence. She may look forward to the opportunity to make new friends, socialize with her hospital roommate, and explore a new environment.
Loss of control	School-age children strive to be independent and productive. They are also greatly influenced by cultural expectations to be "brave and strong" or "grown-up." Hospitalization, which forces the child into a dependent role in an unfamiliar environment, makes it very difficult for the child to continue to meet these goals. She also fears the unknown, such as the possibility of a physical disability or even death. Restrictions on her activities are unwelcome. Feelings of boredom, frustration, anger, and hostility are common reactions to such stressors.
Bodily injury and pain	The school-age child's developing understanding of her body and its functions, together with her growing awareness of her physical capabilities, lead her to feel a higher degree of concern about the impact her illness or injury will have on her lifestyle. She may ask many questions about the permanence of an illness or injury, about limitations imposed on her by the illness or injury, about changes in physical appearance caused by the illness or injury or by medical or surgical treatment, or about the possibility that she will die. She may ask questions about a procedure that will be done, such as whether or not it will hurt, why it has to be done, and what will happen if it does not work. She may refuse a procedure if she fears its negative effects more than she believes in or under-

stands its benefits. Children facing surgery may be afraid that once they are anesthetized, or "put to sleep," they will never wake up. Such fears are largely based on previous exposure to a particular subject. For example, negative experiences that friends or family members have had with medical or surgical treatment may frighten the child into refusing similar treatment. The media and the opinions of peers also will influence the child's view and may result in misunderstandings about the illness, injury, or treatment.

In older children, increased concern for privacy may cause the child to refuse to be examined or have procedures performed in the genital area.

Children's reactions to pain are generally controlled by the age of 9 or 10 years. The child probably will try to behave in what she considers to be a brave manner, suppressing overt reactions to the pain. She may manage the pain by remaining rigid and clenching her teeth or by holding tightly to an object or someone's hand. Some children may want to perform a potentially painful procedure themselves in an effort to control the amount of pain. This may include giving one's own insulin injection, loosening the tape on bandages, or washing a cut. Other children may prefer to be distracted by the television or a video game, requesting that the procedure be done quickly to "get it over with." Still other children will try to avoid the procedure for as long as possible, saying such things as, "Let me finish this game first." In any case, most children are more cooperative about and less fearful of the event when it has been explained to them first.

Coping Strategies

Younger school-age children may want a parent to be with them during medical procedures and as much as possible otherwise, both in the hospital and while recovering at home. Ask the hospital staff if you can be with the child during medical procedures. If you are allowed to be present, give emotional support to the child by holding her hand or by verbally encouraging her. Do not try to assist with the procedure, especially if it is a painful one. The child looks to you for comfort, security, and protection. Your involvement in hurting her will confuse her and weaken her trust in you. Your role should be to comfort the child during and after procedures.

An older child may want more privacy and may not want a caregiver or parent constantly present. Question the child about her preference and be understanding and respectful of her needs. You can show your concern for the child's health and check on her progress by calling her on the bedside telephone, if available, rather than by maintaining a constant vigil at her bedside.

Assist the child with feelings of loneliness and boredom by providing her with appropriate schoolwork and other things to do. Encourage her friends to call or write to her to keep her updated about school activities. Encourage the child to talk about her feelings, and let her know that you recognize she has needs that are not being met. Help her realize that her feelings are normal. It is also important to clarify any misunderstandings she may have about events that have occurred.

You can help the child regain a sense of control by allowing her to make some choices about her care, as her condition permits. Time not allotted to treatments, procedures, diagnostic tests, medications, or meals should be considered the child's free time. Allow the child to plan times for bathing, schoolwork, playing, socializing, watching television, and taking a nap, reinforcing the idea that she has some control over when her daily needs will be met. It may be tempting to sympathize with an ill or injured child and remove all expectations of her in an effort to reduce her burden. This is understandable when a child is critically ill. However, as the child recovers, a drastic change in the role of her parents or in her relationship with them can be very confusing and function especially difficult. Consultation with counselors experienced in working with children, and with families who have dealt with a similar crisis, is usually helpful in gaining support, knowledge, and understanding. It is extremely important to allow the child to work through her feelings as she faces the loss of something she once had. She may be angry and hostile and may resent everyone who tries to help her. She also may resent others, especially her friends, for being able to do what she cannot.

With disability or disfigurement, there may be a period of depression and withdrawal. The child needs time, patience, support, understanding, and encouragement to gain the confidence and motivation she will need to recover. A younger child often does not understand the consequences of a disability and therefore does not grieve such a loss to the degree that an older child does. The younger child is more likely to adapt to the change more quickly as she tries to continue to do what she always has done but in new, imaginative ways. Resenting physical restriction, most children learn how to get around on crutches, in a cast, or in a wheelchair very quickly. The desire to resume their prior levels of activity, independence, and productivity is their prime motivating factor in working toward recovery.

Inform the child's nurse when you feel the child is experiencing pain. Children may not admit they feel pain, sometimes because they fear they will receive an injection. Most pain medications are given intravenously or by mouth, so reassure the child that the medicine will hurt only a little bit or not at all, and that it will help her feel better. Nurses often rely on parents to interpret nonverbal cues indicating that the child needs something, especially with a child who is quiet, shy, or attempting to be brave.

You can also relieve the child's pain by helping her relax through the use of deep breathing. Show the child how to inhale a deep breath of air through her nose, hold it for 2 seconds, and then blow it out slowly and completely through pursed lips, as if blowing out birthday candles. Repeat this several times. Deep breathing helps muscles relax, which can help relieve pain. In addition, focusing the child's attention on breathing rather than on the pain helps her cope with it better. For this reason, distraction through such activities as playing a game, coloring or drawing, working with clay, or watching television is also helpful.

Adolescents (13–19 Years)

Stressors	Behavioral reactions
Separation	The adolescent separated from his peers by hospitalization is likely to feel threatened by a loss of group status and similarity to the group. He does not want to feel that he is different from his peers or inferior in any way. The adolescent may react to separation from peers by withdrawing from interaction with others or by displaying signs of depression, loneliness, and boredom. He may, on the other hand, actually welcome separation from parents and other family members and may view hospitalization as an opportunity to be free from parental restrictions temporarily. Many adolescents also are eager to socialize with new friends they meet during their hospital stay.
Loss of control (loss of identity, enforced dependency)	The adolescent stage of human development marks a transition from childhood to adulthood. During this time, the adolescent strives to establish a separate identity. He wants to be independent and to be able to make his own decisions about issues that affect his lifestyle. Hospitalization may force him back into the dependent role he has been struggling to abandon. Physical limitations may require him to be dependent on others for

may deprive him of the opportunity to make his own decisions about daily activities. Many adolescents react negatively to this new role and reject others, withdraw from interaction with others, or refuse to cooperate with hospital staff or family members in aspects of their care. They may display unusual anger, frustration, and assertiveness, and may even become demanding at times.

The adolescent fears the unknown and may ask many questions about his treatment. He wants to have some control over his condition, and may request that he be allowed to participate in a procedure, such as removing his bandage, administering his breathing treatment, taking his temperature, and so on.

Bodily injury and pain

Concern with body image is of paramount importance during the adolescent years. An adolescent's perception of the severity of an illness or injury is most often based on his fear of the effect it will have on his bodily appearance and on his ability to carry on a lifestyle similar to that of peers. The adolescent already feels insecure about his body because of the normal physical changes he is experiencing, and so any threat to this image is a major concern.

The adolescent may fear the effect that medical or surgical treatment will have on his body and may refuse surgery or other treatments that will cause changes in physical appearance or impose physical limitations. He may refuse to cooperate in his treatment and may question the adequacy and appropriateness of his care. He may withdraw from or reject others.

The adolescent attempts to react to pain with significant self-control. He typically does not display the resistant behavior of the younger child when a painful procedure is to be performed. In some cases, the adolescent may want to benefit from being sick, especially given the attention it can bring. His complaints of pain must be doctors and nurses and ask them to more fully explain the rationale for, and details of, tests or procedures. The adolescent usually will be much more cooperative and consenting if he has been informed about a procedure in advance, especially if he has been allowed to participate in some of the decision making surrounding the procedure.

Since the adolescent's acceptance by his peer group is so important to him, any physical disability or disfigurement, whether temporary or permanent, can be devastating to his self-esteem. He will need a great deal of emotional support and encouragement from family and friends. Consultation with counselors experienced in working with adolescents, and with adolescents and families who have dealt with a similar crisis, is usually helpful in gaining support, knowledge, and understanding.

With disability or disfigurement, there may be a period of depression and withdrawal. The child needs time to work through his feelings as he faces the loss of something he used to have. He may be angry and hostile and may resent everyone who tries to help him. He also may resent others, especially siblings or friends, for being able to do what he cannot. Allow him to have these feelings while also focusing on other existing or newly learned capabilities. It is important for the child to have hope and a positive outlook to gain the confidence and motivation he will need to work toward recovery.

Pain relief may be necessary to promote the child's recovery, especially since he may be exerting himself by participating in physical therapy and routine self-care activities. The adolescent does not usually fear the administration of pain medication. In fact, many adolescents enjoy the euphoric feeling afforded by some medications. This is especially true of adolescents who habitually use alcohol or other drugs or who are experiencing depression or a drastic adjustment due to illness or injury.

It is important to distinguish between a sincere need for pain relief and a desire for the mental effects of pain medication.

You can also relieve the child's pain by helping him relax through the use of deep breathing. Show the child how to inhale a deep breath of air through his nose, hold it for 2 seconds, and then blow it out slowly and completely through pursed lips. Deep breathing helps muscles relax, which can help relieve pain. The adolescent may not be very cooperative in a teaching session, but he may use this deep-breathing technique at a later time. Meditation is also an effective pain reliever, and may be appropriate for some adolescents. Books on meditation techniques are available at most libraries. Distraction through other activities is also helpful for pain relief. Provide the child with books, magazines, games, stationery, music, and even "dreaded" schoolwork.

American Academy of Orthopaedic Surgeons. *Emergency Care and Transportation of the Sick and Injured.* Chicago: American Academy of Orthopaedic Surgeons, 1971.

American Heart Association and American Academy of Pediatrics. *Textbook of Pediatric Basic Life Support.* Dallas, Texas: American Heart Association, 1988.

American Medical Association. "Guidelines for Cardiopulmonary Resuscitation and Emergency Cardiac Care: Recommendations of the 1992 National Conference." *The Journal of the American Medical Association,* October 28, 1992, p. 2251.

American Red Cross. *American Red Cross: Basic Rescue and Water Safety.* New York: American National Red Cross, 1980.

———. *Multimedia Standard First Aid.* Steamboat Springs, Colorado: American National Red Cross, 1987.

———. *Standard First Aid and Personal Safety,* 2d ed. New York: Doubleday and Company, Inc., 1979.

Burman, A.M., et al. *Advanced Skills in Emergency Care: A Text for the Intermediate EMT.* Akron, Ohio: American Academy of Orthopaedic Surgeons, 1982.

deToledo, L. W. "Infant CPR: Do You Know What to Do?" *Canadian Nurse,* May 1984, p. 44.

Eisenberg, M., et al. "Epidemiology of Cardiac Arrest and Resuscitation in Children." *Annals of Emergency Medicine,* November 1983, p. 672.

Guzy, P.M., et al. "The Survival Benefit of Bystander Cardiopulmonary Resuscitation in a Paramedic Served Metropolitan Area." *American Journal of Public Health,* July 1983, pp. 766–768.

Kravitz, H. "Accident Prevention Research." *Pediatric Annals,* January 1973, pp. 47–53.

Levine, M.I. "A Pediatrician's View." *Pediatric Annals,* January 1973, pp. 5–6.

Martin, T.G. "Near Drowning and Cold Water Immersion." *Annals of Emergency Medicine,* April 1984, pp. 263–273.

McKenna, S. "Changing Behavior Towards Danger: The Effect of First Aid Training." *Journal of Occupational Accidents,* April 1982, pp. 47–59.

McKenna, S., and S. Blaylock. "First Aid and Home Safety Training in the Community." *Occupational Health,* March 1983, pp. 122–129.

Pantell, R.H., M.D., et al. *Taking Care of Your Child.* Reading, Massachusetts: Addison-Wesley Publishing Company, 1984.

Scipien, G., et al. *Comprehensive Pediatric Nursing.* New York: McGraw-Hill Book Company, 1975.

Whaley, L.F., and D.L. Wong. *Nursing Care of Infants and Children.* St. Louis: C.V. Mosby Company, 1979.

Wheatley, G. "Childhood Accidents 1952–1972: An Overview." *Pediatric Annals,* January 1973, p. 10.